DATE DUE

NOV 1 4 2016		
NOV 1 2 2018		
DEC 1 7 2018		
		PRINTED IN U.S.A.

THE BIG SQUEEZE

A VOLUME IN THE SERIES

The Culture and Politics
of Health Care Work

edited by
SUZANNE GORDON AND SIOBAN NELSON

A list of titles in this series is available
at www.cornellpress.cornell.edu.

HANDEL REYNOLDS, MD

THE BIG

A Social and Political History of the

Controversial Mammogram

SQUEEZE

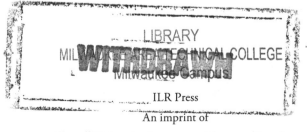

ILR Press

An imprint of

Cornell University Press • Ithaca and London

First published 2012 by Cornell University Press
Printed in the United States of America

Library of Congress Cataloging-in-Publication Data

Reynolds, Handel, 1963–
    The big squeeze : a social and political history of the controversial mammogram / Handel Reynolds.
        p. cm. — (The culture and politics of health care work)
    Includes bibliographical references and index.
    ISBN 978-0-8014-5093-8 (cloth : alk. paper)
    1. Breast—Radiography—United States—History. 2. Breast—Cancer—Diagnosis—United States—History. I. Title. II. Series: Culture and politics of health care work.
    RG493.5.R33R49 2012
    618.1'90754—dc23   2012013738

Cloth printing   10 9 8 7 6 5 4 3 2 1

To my dear family, Marlene, Gevin, and Telissa

for their unfailing love and support

CONTENTS

THE BIG SQUEEZE

INTRODUCTION

The Mammography Story

The story cried out to be told. It cried out in the passion of the true believers, apologists for a beleaguered test. It cried out in the polemics of the skeptics, emphasizing possible risks and advising caution. It cried out in the posturing of political leaders who co-opted a scientific debate to satisfy the expediency of the moment. It cried out in the gratitude and calm resignation of those for whom mammography worked. And it cried out in the silent pain and anguish of those who did "everything right," yet for whom mammography failed.

Over the years, our national conversation on mammography has often resembled the ancient Indian parable of the blind men and the elephant. In this tale, each man feels just one of the animal's body parts and tries to describe the essence of the beast. Thus, one feels the elephant's sturdy leg and declares, "The elephant is much like a pillar." Another feels its thin tail and concludes, "The elephant is much like a rope," and so on. This book attempts to take a step back, remove the blinders, and tell the whole story.

From the beginning, mammography has been promoted as a silver bullet in the fight against breast cancer, the most important thing a woman can do to "protect" herself from the dreaded disease. This "mammogram protector" metaphor has been a dominant theme in public education campaigns throughout the history of the test. It has been very successful in establishing a culture of screening. Yet this simplistic rendition of a complex issue has also had many undesirable effects. Most important, it has contributed to a pervasive misunderstanding of what mammography is and what it does. Many women overestimate mammography's capabilities; others confuse *screening* with *prevention*. Thus, not surprisingly, anger and confusion are common responses when a woman is diagnosed with breast cancer despite faithfully undergoing annual testing.

Mammography has been mired in controversy since its earliest days. The question whether women under fifty should be screened first became a contentious debate in 1976, only three years after its nationwide debut. This dispute has dogged mammography throughout its existence, becoming more acrimonious with each eruption. There are two reasons for this. The first is that the debate has never been entirely about science. In this book I show that major stakeholders in this debate—namely, the American Cancer Society and the American College of Radiology—adopted a "pro" position on this question, long before there was any scientific basis for it. In the ensuing decades, it has become clear that the science supporting screening is much more robust for women over fifty (postmenopausal) than for younger women. Thus, in most of the developed world, public health policy calls for screening to begin at age fifty. In the United States, the backers of under-fifty screening succeeded by convincing political leaders that it was expedient to be on the "right" side of this issue. In taking that position, they would demonstrate appropriate sensitivity to women's health issues. As this occurred, the nexus of the debate moved from the realm of science to politics. Here it has resided, at least since the mid-1990s. The second reason why the screening of women younger than fifty is mammography's perennial dispute is that both parties in this argument claim to have science on their side. Because there is some scientific justification for both positions, each side has taken to denouncing studies that conflict with its view and highlighting those that support it. Thus, over time, positions have become more rigid and uncompromising.

Now more than ever, women deserve an open and frank discussion of mammography, its benefits, and its potential risks. Not only does the controversy regarding under-fifty screening continue unabated, but also there is a growing body of research that questions whether decades of screening mammography has accomplished anything at all. These studies suggest that the observed reduction in the death rate from breast cancer is due to improvements in treatment rather than early detection. As we approach the fortieth anniversary of the start of widespread screening mammography in the United States, it is a fitting time to pause and reflect.

The Big Squeeze: A Social and Political History of the Controversial Mammogram chronicles the often turbulent history of screening mammography since its introduction in the early 1970s. This book makes five key points. First, it shows how pivotal decisions during mammography's initial roll-out made it all but inevitable that the test would never be far from controversy. Second, it describes how, at several key points in its history, the establishment of a culture of mammography screening was greatly aided by concurrent social and political forces and movements. Third, it illustrates how politics came to dominate the debate, eventually achieving primacy over science itself. Fourth, *The Big Squeeze* describes the collateral economy that developed around screening. As mammography was aggressively promoted in the late 1980s to early 1990s, utilization rates rapidly increased. As this occurred, the mundane mammogram became the little *pink* engine that could, and did, drive the growth of a vast screening-dependent secondary economy. Finally, mammography's burden, overdiagnosis, is considered in the last chapter. Overdiagnosis, the screening detection of cancers that would never otherwise have come to light in the individual's lifetime, is an important yet woefully underdiscussed risk of mammography. This phenomenon is more significant than that, however. Overdiagnosis helped make fighting breast cancer the most favored disease cause and mammography the most favored weapon in the fight.

The story of mammography fascinates me for several reasons. First, no other medical test even comes close in the degree of passion and controversy it evokes. Between the true believers and the skeptics, the mammography debates of the past four decades have showcased the full range of human emotion. Second, no medical test has been so completely "adopted" by political leaders eager to demonstrate their sensitivity to women's issues. They have not simply appropriated the debate, however; they have largely converted it from a scientific to a political one. Finally, and this may be the most fascinating point of all, the central argument in the disputes over mammography—namely, whether or not women under fifty should be screened—hasn't changed in the entire forty-year history of the test. As a radiologist, I have witnessed the unfolding of this compelling history firsthand. Through *The Big Squeeze*, I wish to share it with you.

First, though, a word about definitions. Throughout this book the term "mammography" should be understood to mean "screening mammography." This is a test that is performed on women without breast-related symptoms or complaints, to search for unsuspected breast cancer. In the United States it is typically performed at one- to two-year intervals on women, starting at age forty. This is the subject of the book. There will be occasional references to "diagnostic mammography." This is mammography used to evaluate a specific problem the patient may have, such as breast pain or a lump. This test is done on an as-needed basis. It is not a central part of this discussion.

(1)

TIMING IS EVERYTHING

Screening mammography burst onto the stage of national consciousness in 1973. When it did, it found an audience primed to receive it. Political, social, and health movements that had been occurring in the larger American society underwent a remarkable convergence in the late 1960s to mid-1970s. This was precisely the time when the results of the earliest medical research on mammography were becoming widely known. Though it is likely that this new screening test would have been successful on its own, this fortuitous alignment of external forces helped ensure that public acceptance would be rapid and durable. In this chapter I examine the three principal movements that set the stage for screening mammography's auspicious debut. In its subsequent history, newer incarnations of these same forces would surface repeatedly, particularly at times of great controversy.

Cancer Fighting as Good Politics

On March 25, 1970, Senator Ralph Yarborough, a Texas Democrat, made an impassioned speech on the floor of the United States

Senate. In it he bemoaned the lack of significant progress toward the eradication of cancer in the thirty-three years since the establishment of the National Cancer Institute (NCI). Yarborough, who had been in the Senate for thirteen years, was a progressive southern Democrat who, as chairman of the Labor and Public Welfare Committee (now the Health, Education, Labor and Pensions Committee), was a frequent and forceful voice on health issues. As he saw it, the cause of this stagnation was twofold. Primarily it was due to severe under-resourcing of the effort. He pointed out that the approximately $200 million per year being spent at the time on the government's anti-cancer efforts was "far less than the $358 million we spend each year for chewing gum."[1] The second was the lack of a clear national focus and determination to accomplish the goal. To Yarborough and like-minded political leaders, the successes of the Manhattan Project and the Apollo program were apt case studies in what was possible when the nation was determined to spare no effort in order to achieve a seemingly impossible goal. Yarborough's conversations with leading cancer experts, notably Sidney Farber, a distinguished Boston oncologist and president of the American Cancer Society (ACS), led him to believe that a major breakthrough in cancer control was imminent. In fact, a few months earlier, at the November 1969 annual meeting of the ACS, Farber had urged a $2 billion a year effort, modeled after the space program, to achieve cancer control. "Without naming the day or year, such a conquest is a realistic goal," he is reported to have said at a press conference.[2] Going much further, Yarborough and forty-six co-sponsors introduced a resolution calling for the creation of a Committee of Consultants on the Conquest of Cancer. The committee was charged with recommending "to Congress and to the American people what must be done to achieve cures for the major forms of cancer by 1976—the 200th anniversary of the founding of this great Republic."[3] The Yarborough resolution was adopted by the full Senate and resulted in the constitution of a twenty-six-member Committee of Consultants, co-chaired by Farber and Benno C. Schmidt, chairman of the board of the trustees of Memorial Hospital in New York.[4]

Nineteen seventy would prove to be Yarborough's last full year in the Senate. In May of that year he was defeated in the Texas Democratic primary election by conservative businessman Lloyd Bentsen Jr. in a particularly bitter political contest.[5] The Committee of Consultants presented part one of its report to the Senate's Labor and Welfare Committee in the fall of 1970. Despite his recent electoral trouncing, Yarborough, in the final days of his Senate service, introduced a major piece of health care legislation. The Conquest of Cancer Act, introduced in December 1970, incorporated most of the major recommendations of the advisory committee. Its primary provision was to call for the establishment of an independent cancer-fighting agency, the National Cancer Authority (modeled after the National Aeronautics and Space Administration), which would take over all the responsibilities of the NCI but would not be a part of the National Institutes of Health.

At the White House the battle was about to be joined. President Richard M. Nixon, sensing that Congress had tapped into an issue likely to resonate with the American people, was not going to miss an opportunity to demonstrate presidential leadership. The public was becoming increasingly frustrated with the Vietnam War, and he was eager to change the subject of the national conversation. In his State of the Union message on January 22, 1971, he called for an extra $100 million appropriation to "launch an intensive campaign to find a cure for cancer." At no previous time in American history had cancer received this level of presidential attention. Nixon went on to declare: "The time has come in America when the same kind of concentrated effort that split the atom and took man to the moon should be turned toward conquering this dread disease. Let us make a total national commitment to achieve this goal."[6]

Competing cancer-fighting bills were introduced and debated in Congress that year. A modified version of the Yarborough bill was introduced by Senator Edward M. Kennedy, a Massachusetts Democrat, and a Nixon-backed bill was proposed by Senator Peter H. Dominick, a Colorado Republican. After a contentious yearlong legislative effort, the National Cancer Act of 1971 was signed into law on December 23. In his signing statement Nixon extended the now familiar military metaphor associated with the anticancer effort. Referring to new presidential powers granted by the act, he vowed that "the President will be able to take personal command of the Federal effort to conquer cancer."[7] Not only would he be commander in chief of a military battling an enemy in Southeast Asia, but also he would be personally leading the charge against an enemy much closer to home. It is in this regard that Nixon is commonly considered to have launched the nation's "War on Cancer," even though, as we have seen, the fight was well under way by the time he arrived on the battlefield.

The National Cancer Act provided massive new federal funding for the country's anticancer effort ($1.6 billion in the first three years) and significantly elevated the status of the NCI. Of all its provisions, however, one in particular, the allocation of $90 million to fund cooperative cancer control programs with state or private agencies, would quickly prove pivotal in the establishment of mammographic screening.[8]

Feminism and Women's Health

The women's health movement of the 1960s and 1970s constitutes the fourth wave of what the sociologist Carol Weisman describes as a larger "mega-movement" in women's health, a phenomenon that began with the women's health component of the popular health movement of the 1830s and 1840s and continued through the women's health political agenda of the early 1990s.[9] Women of the baby boom generation entered the period of peak reproductive potential in the 1960s, and it was these women, primarily in their twenties and thirties, who were the leaders of this movement.[10] Not surprisingly, their primary concern was asserting control over their reproductive functions. This movement, which was intertwined with the feminist movement of the same period, was motivated by a viewpoint which held that women did not have ultimate control over their own bodies and their own health.[11] As noted by Sheryl Ruzek, author of a detailed history of this movement, "from the Supreme Court to the examining room, men were making fateful decisions about women's bodies and their reproductive lives."[12] Abortion was illegal in most states, and many had laws limiting the sale and distribution of contraceptives. To further its goal of reordering the balance of power between the male-dominated medical and political establishments and the masses of laywomen, the women's health movement employed two main strategies: self-help groups and political action organizations.[13] The Boston Women's Health Book Collective, the most famous of the self-help groups, consisted of a group of laywomen who met regularly to commiserate about their feelings of "frustration, and anger toward . . . the medical [system and] . . . doctors who were condescending, paternalistic, judgmental and non-informative."[14] The groundbreaking self-help women's health manual *Our Bodies, Ourselves* was published by this group in 1971. It presented detailed information, all of it obtained through the painstaking research of group members, on topics such as contraception, abortion, the female sexual response, and sexually transmitted disease, to an audience of women unaccustomed to frank treatment of such subjects. The self-help gynecology movement, begun in April 1971 by the feminist Carol Downer, taught women how to perform a speculum examination on themselves or other women.[15] Self-help groups in Chicago formed a network of facilities (known simply as "Jane") where laywomen provided safe (illegal) abortion services.[16] Freestanding birthing centers and the concept of "natural" childbirth took root in various parts of the country as a response to what many women saw as the "medicalization" of childbirth.[17]

Important accomplishments of the women's health movement during this time include the Supreme Court decisions *Griswold v. Connecticut* (1965), which invalidated a Connecticut law that made it illegal for married couples to obtain or use contraceptives, and *Roe v. Wade* (1973), which invalidated a Texas law banning abortion, legalizing the procedure nationwide for the first time.

According to Weisman, "the Women's Health Movement created a cohort of women concerned about matters of health and health care and a network of organizations to sustain this activism."[18] Although in the 1960s and 1970s the issue for these twenty- and thirty-year-old baby boomers was reproductive health, it was this same cohort of activist women, primed and ready for action, who would fight the mammography and breast cancer battles as forty- and fifty-year-olds in the late 1980s and early 1990s.[19]

Preaching the Gospel of Early Detection

For most of the twentieth century, the principal theme of public discourse on breast cancer was early detection. This arose from the prevailing medical view of cancer as, initially, a local disease that, if treated early and aggressively, could be cured. As early as 1894, William Halsted, the renowned Johns Hopkins University surgeon who pioneered the radical mastectomy, wrote that "cancer of the breast is a curable disease if operated upon properly and in time."[20] Whether by design or happenstance, Halsted's phrase "operated upon properly and in time" encapsulated the essence of the cancer education programs that would come to dominate the new century. The point was simply that surgery cures cancer, but *only* if the patient presents to the surgeon promptly. A May 1913 *Ladies' Home Journal* article titled "What Can We Do about Cancer?" put it bluntly: "No cancer is hopeless when discovered early. Most cancer, discovered early, is curable. The only cure is the knife. Medicines are worse than useless. Delay is more than dangerous; it is deadly. The one hope, and a strong one, is prompt and radical operation; a half operation is worse than none at all."[21]

Founded in 1913 by a group of surgeons, the American Society for the Control of Cancer (ASCC) was warmly received and fully endorsed by the larger medical establishment. From its inception, the dominant message of the ASCC was that surgeons could effectively treat (and cure) cancer in its earliest stages.[22] Early on, cancers specific to women received particular attention. To reach the female public more effectively, the male-dominated ASCC established an all-female wing, the Women's Field Army, in 1937. This organization, modeled after a military unit down to the military-style uniforms and insignia its members wore, became known as the "educational arm of the ASCC."[23] At its peak, the Women's Field Army had 700,000 members, each having paid a one-time enrollment fee of one dollar.[24] These large funds were used to finance a massive public education campaign consisting of mass meetings, lectures, radio broadcasts, and newspaper and magazine articles, as well as educational brochures. Women were the target audience, and the focus was breast and reproductive cancers.[25] The overall message was threefold: that cancer could be cured, that early detection allowed successful treatment, and that regular medical checkups for women, even when they were feeling well, were essential.[26]

In 1944 the ASCC underwent a major restructuring incited by a prominent New York philanthropist and health care activist, Mary Lasker. In addition to a change in the governance of the organization, the ASCC was rebranded the American Cancer Society. Shortly thereafter the Women's Field Army was integrated into the ACS and the organization adopted a new focus: securing funds for cancer research through charitable donations. Its initial fund-raising activities were wildly successful, and within its first year of existence the ACS became the largest nongovernmental funding agency for cancer research.[27]

Promoting early detection, however, remained a major focus of the ACS. In 1948 it produced, *Life Saving Fingers*, the first educational film on breast self-examination (BSE). In it, a woman, undressed from the waist up, demonstrated the procedure. The film was narrated by Dr. Alfred Popma, a Boise, Idaho, radiologist who is credited with developing the first educational materials specifically describing the proper technique for BSE.[28] It was widely distributed and shown to packed houses in major cinemas.[29]

In addition to films, the postwar period saw continued dissemination of the early detection message in articles and advertisements in the popular press, posters, and educational pamphlets. As noted by the historian Kirsten Gardner, many of these directly targeted women and used fictional characters who demonstrated "good/wise" or "bad/foolish" behavior by following or not following ACS recommendations for early detection.[30] A "wise" woman was one who noted a lump in her breast and quickly sought treatment. She was portrayed as happy and healthy. A "foolish" woman ignored her lump, not seeking care until it was too late. She was portrayed as depressed and dying. Thus, observes Gardner, "women's behavior became the key variable in cancer control. . . . [I]f a woman with cancer failed to follow early detection principles, death seemed inevitable, and the victim assumed the blame."[31] There was little to no discussion of the difficulty and uncertainty inherent in examining breasts (limitations of early detection), the physical impact of radical mastectomy (the only treatment available at the time), or the possibility that death may still occur despite "wise" behavior (treatment failure). While this single-minded focus on early detection may have been well intentioned, calculated to empower women and replace fear with hope, it had unintended consequences, some of which still echo faintly today in the guilt many women experience when a cancerous lump is found by their doctor or on a mammogram—guilt for having "failed" at BSE by not finding it first.

At this point it is helpful to digress briefly and consider another important female reproductive cancer. The American Cancer Society's efforts against cervical cancer would come to define its approach to screening mammography some decades later.

In January 1928 George Papanicolaou, a Greek-born pathologist who had emigrated to the United States in 1913, presented some preliminary observations at the Third Race Betterment Conference in Battle Creek, Michigan.[32] Papanicolaou, working at Cornell Medical College,[33] had obtained daily vaginal smears from a group of women and examined them microscopically for cellular aberrations. He showed that malignant cells and precancerous lesions could be detected with this simple technique. Papanicolaou's work aroused very little interest in the medical community for many years. Surgical orthodoxy at the time accepted open biopsy[34] as the only reliable means of diagnosing cervical cancer. In the 1930s and 1940s Papanicolaou's findings were reproduced by other researchers, yet there was limited adoption of the new technique. Major barriers to adopting the Pap test were lack of education among physicians and the lay public as well as absence of an infrastructure of professional cytotechnicians and pathologists trained in the technique.

With these considerations in mind, an ambitious five-year cervical cancer screening program was launched in 1952. Dubbed the Memphis Project, it was jointly sponsored by the Cancer Control Branch of the NCI, the University of Tennessee, and the Memphis branch of the ACS. The goal of the project was to screen all 165,000 women over the age of twenty in the Memphis–Shelby County, Tennessee, area annually for five years.[35] The ACS and its army of volunteers played an important role in the public education component of the project.[36] During the course of the study, over 150,000 women were screened, and a large number of early stage cervical cancers were diagnosed. Prior to the initiation of screening, 34 percent of white and 18 percent of African American cervical cancer patients in the Memphis–Shelby County area were diagnosed in stage 1. During the program, these rates increased to 57 percent and 38 percent, respectively.[37]

The success of the Memphis Project showed that the Pap smear could be efficiently applied to large populations, that early detection of cervical cancer was possible, and thus lives could be saved.[38] In 1953 the U.S. death rate from uterine cancer (including cancer of the cervix as well as the body of the uterus) was 16.8 per 100,000 women. By 1963 the death rate had been reduced by a remarkable 27 percent, to 12.2 per 100,000.[39] This notable achievement was largely due to widespread adoption of the Pap smear in routine gynecologic care. The Pap smear represents the most dramatic validation of early detection in the history of medicine. These efforts were viewed as unmitigated triumphs of the principles long espoused by the ACS. The elixir of success strengthened its resolve and bolstered its confidence.

Thus, by the time screening mammography was introduced to the public in the early 1970s, the notion of early detection for effective cancer control had been successfully inculcated in the American psyche. The new screening test promised to be more reliable than the patient's fingers and would lighten the burden that self-examination placed upon her. The ACS, hoping to reproduce its success against cervical cancer, would again play a leading role in the dissemination of a new screening technology. Add to this the new cancer-fighting political agenda in Washington, D.C., and the growing women's health care activism, and the stage was set for screening mammography to have a successful opening act.

(2)

FIRST EXPOSURE

In medicine, the introduction of new imaging technology is typically a three-phase process.[1] In the first phase, diffusion occurs slowly as early adopters—academics and other "technology leaders"— perform much of the initial clinical research that defines the capability of the new device. If these results are favorable, then as they are disseminated in medical journals and professional conferences, there comes a point when a rapid increase in the adoption of the new technology is observed. This second phase is often aided by media attention, which in turn drives consumer interest. Finally, as market saturation is achieved, the rate of diffusion levels off.

Mammography's path was not so orderly or predictable. In 1970 the age-adjusted death rate from breast cancer in the United States stood at approximately 27 per 100,000 women, essentially unchanged since record keeping began in 1930.[2] All the efforts of the first half of the twentieth century, promoting early detection and prompt radical surgery, had accomplished very little. When the American Cancer Society launched the massive Breast Cancer Detection Demonstration Project (BCDDP) in 1973, most Americans had never heard of mammography. Their first exposure would be a crash course.

The BCDDP: A New Screening
Regimen Emerges

Mammography was not new in 1973. Like the Pap smear, it had languished through a prolonged season of indifference. Clinical mammography (that is, on live patients) was first reported by Stafford Warren in 1930.[3] In the 1930s and 1940s there were sporadic other reports of clinical mammography in the medical literature. These all described using X-ray to examine the breasts of patients who were already suspected of having breast cancer because of the presence of a lump or other symptoms. High-quality images were very difficult to obtain, however, and the technique was hard to reproduce outside select research institutions. Mammography never caught on.

Interest in mammography was renewed as a result of two important developments that occurred in 1960–61. In 1961, the radiologist Jacob Gershon-Cohen, of Albert Einstein Medical Center in Philadelphia, reported on his findings from mammography in healthy women (that is, with no physical signs or symptoms of breast cancer). In 1956 he had recruited 1,312 such women, who then underwent mammography and physical examination every six months for five years. During the course of the study, twenty-three cancers were discovered, six of which could not be palpated on physical examination but were identified solely on the basis of the mammographic findings.[4] This study was significant for two important reasons: it was the first use of mammography as a screening tool (that is, to evaluate women who had no suspicion of breast cancer), and it was one of the first demonstrations that mammography could identify breast cancer that could not be felt by a surgeon.

At about the same time that Gershon-Cohen was initiating his screening study in Philadelphia, another radiologist, Robert Egan, was completing his radiology training at M. D. Anderson Cancer Center in Houston. His department chairman had assigned him the task of solving the technical problems of mammography. By varying the intensity and quantity of the radiation used, as well as experimenting with a variety of different X-ray film types, Egan's work produced the technical breakthrough that mammography needed. When he published his results in 1960, he described the technical factors required to produce high-quality mammograms reliably. Using his technique, one thousand mammograms were performed on women suspected of having breast cancer. Not only was he able to identify correctly 238 of 240 known malignant tumors, but also he identified 19 tumors in breasts that were thought to be normal on the basis of the surgeon's physical examination.[5]

As an aside, it should be noted that at this stage in its history, mammography was performed with general purpose X-ray equipment, such as might be used to X-ray a broken bone. Machines designed specifically for mammography, such as we have today, were not introduced in the United States until 1967, when the French medical equipment manufacturer CGR unveiled the Senograph. By the early 1970s, there were multiple manufacturers selling similar *dedicated* mammography machines.[6] The practice of using general purpose X-ray equipment for mammography did not completely disappear, however, until the late 1980s.

In the mid-1960s, the U.S. Public Health Service undertook a study in which radiologists from twenty-four institutions around the country went to M. D. Anderson to learn the Egan technique and were then observed to see if they could reproduce it in their own institutions. The results showed that the technique was highly reproducible.[7]

The momentum was building. In 1962 Dr. Philip Strax, director of radiology at City Hospital in New York, approached the leadership of the Health Insurance Plan (HIP) of Greater New York, a private health insurance company, with the results of Gershon-Cohen's and Egan's work.[8] Strax, whose first wife, Bertha, had died of breast cancer at age thirty-nine, was very passionate about the disease. He had studied the Egan technique and had been offering mammography as part of his practice. He felt strongly that the time had come for a large, carefully designed study of the effectiveness of mammography as a screening test for breast cancer. Coincidentally, the National Cancer Institute was interested in funding such a study and was looking for a suitable site.[9]

The HIP mammography trial began in 1963. It was directed by Strax; Sam Shapiro, an internist with the HIP research and statistics department; and Louis Venet, a surgeon at New York Medical College. In this study, 62,000 women between the ages of forty and sixty-four were randomly assigned to one of two groups. The screening group received mammography and physical examination at enrollment and at three subsequent annual follow-up visits. The mammography was a modification of the Egan technique. The control group received only the usual medical care, which at the time did not include routine mammography. The results, reported in the *Journal of the American Medical Association* in March 1971, were dramatic.[10] After three and a half years of follow-up, there were 40 percent fewer breast cancer deaths among women aged fifty to fifty-nine who were in the screening group than among those in the control group. Furthermore, 70 percent of women who had their cancer diagnosed by screening had no disease in their lymph nodes, compared to 45 percent in the control group, indicating that screening caught the disease earlier, before it had spread. Finally, of the 127 confirmed breast cancers in the screening group, 42 (33 percent) were found by mammography alone.

The HIP trial was the first scientific validation of the concept of mammographic screening. At this writing it remains the only mammography study of its kind (a randomized controlled trial) ever performed in the United States. It is important to note that the benefits of screening were seen only in women fifty to fifty-nine years old. No benefit was demonstrated for women sixty to sixty-four or forty to forty-nine. These limitations did not dampen the enthusiasm with which the results were greeted when they were presented at the American Cancer Society's Second National Conference on Breast Cancer in Los Angeles in May 1971.[11] To the ACS, it was starting to feel like Memphis all over again.

It was sometime shortly thereafter that Philip Strax approached ACS Vice President for Medical Affairs Dr. Arthur Holleb with a bold vision of an ACS-sponsored nationwide program of free screening mammography.[12] Not needing much convincing, the ACS board of directors formally endorsed Strax's vision in February 1972.[13] The Breast Cancer Detection Demonstration Project, in its original version, called for the establishment of twelve individual detection projects, three in each of the four ACS administrative divisions (East, South, Midwest, and West). Each was to enroll ten thousand healthy women, aged thirty-five to seventy-four, for free annual screening consisting of physical examination, mammography, thermography (a technology based on sensing temperature differences in various parts of the breast as means of identifying cancer),[14] and instruction in breast self-examination.[15] A budget of $2 million was established to fund the program for two years. With the recent signing of the National Cancer Act, large sums of federal funds, designated for cancer control programs, were ready to be disbursed. Perceiving an opportunity to do something on a truly grand scale, in 1972 the ACS formally proposed to the National Cancer Institute that the BCDDP be a jointly sponsored program.[16] The new NCI-ACS demonstration project was to be the first major cancer control program in the nation's new War on Cancer.[17] Its reach was more than doubled, to twenty-seven geographic locations (two sites ran two detection projects each, for a total of twenty-nine individual projects), and its budget tripled to $6 million, with the ACS providing one third and the NCI two thirds. With the dramatic increase in the proposed number of centers, the number of expected participants grew to 280,000, and the period of screening was increased to five years.

The decisions to perform a demonstration project, as opposed to a true research trial, and to screen women as young as thirty-five years old have been widely debated in the decades since the BCDDP. A demonstration project is typically undertaken once the scientific validity of the intervention (here, screening mammography) has been firmly established.[18] It is done to show how a test of proven value may be widely implemented. At the time, the only scientific validation of screening mammography was the HIP trial, and it had shown benefit only for women in the fifty to fifty-nine age group. It is clear that the main goal of the effort was simply to demonstrate that mass population screening with mammography was feasible and practical.[19] It is also clear that some NCI scientists had misgivings about the lack of a scientific orientation to the BCDDP.[20] Women thirty-five to forty-nine years old were recruited for screening despite the absence of evidence that screening would benefit them. The sense of the ACS was that if screening worked for women fifty to fifty-nine, it would probably work for women of all ages, so its use should not be restricted. Recalling the early days of the program, Arthur Holleb, chief medical officer of the ACS from 1968 to 1988, noted in a 1992 article, "The HIP study showed an early benefit of screening in women beginning at 50 years of age, but the . . . American Cancer Society believed that the BCDDP should begin screening at age 35 years of age because more years of life might be saved."[21] One can only surmise that Philip Strax's own experience of losing his wife to breast cancer at such a young age helped inform this decision.

The first three BCDDP centers were designated in January 1973, and by February 1974, all twenty-seven had been publicly announced.[22] By the time the first patients were screened in July 1973, the ACS had already mobilized its vast nationwide army of volunteers, numbering 2.5 million at the time.[23] This massive effort was run out of local ACS chapter offices and involved working with women's clubs as well as utilizing radio, television, and newspaper advertising. As with all successful grass-roots campaigns, it was the person-to-person contact that proved most effective. Forty-four percent of BCDDP participants stated that they had heard about the program from a friend, as opposed to 29 percent from the newspaper, 11 percent from television, and 9 percent from their physician.[24] By early 1974 there were reports of sites receiving two hundred telephone calls per day from women eager to participate. Nationally, appointment wait times grew to between three and six weeks.[25]

In the fall of 1974 the BCDDP received an unexpected boost. On September 28 President Gerald Ford, at the conclusion of an economics conference, announced to the nation that his wife, Betty, had been diagnosed with breast cancer and had just undergone a radical mastectomy.[26] The tumor in Mrs. Ford's right breast had been found during a routine medical checkup days before. She would later credit early detection for her excellent prognosis. Approximately three weeks later, on October 18, Vice President–designate Nelson Rockefeller disclosed that his forty-eight-year-old wife, Margaretta (Happy), had undergone a mastectomy the previous day.[27] Mrs. Rockefeller had identified a lump in her left breast on self-examination two weeks earlier. Rockefeller stated that his wife's recognition of the lump had been aided by a "heightened consciousness" following Mrs. Ford's surgery.[28] The lump was confirmed by a visit to her gynecologist, who ordered additional testing, including a mammogram.

While neither Betty Ford nor Happy Rockefeller had her breast cancer detected by a *screening* mammogram, the intense media attention surrounding their diagnoses caused a surge in interest in mammography. BCDDP centers and non-BCDDP mammography facilities were overwhelmed with women demanding a mammogram. This intensified interest extended even beyond the usual demographics. College women, on the advice of campus health officials, began undergoing screening mammography in large numbers.[29]

Significantly aided by this Ford-Rockefeller effect, the BCDDP completed the initial round of screening on 270,000 women in the first two years of the program.[30] As a result of this spike in screening rates, there was a 14 percent increase in the incidence of breast cancer in the United States during 1974–75. Those were the heady early days of mammography. The new screening test had rapidly achieved widespread public acceptance. There was a fresh sense of optimism about the potential of modern medical technology to conquer breast cancer. Mammography's "new car smell" would not last long, however. Already the faint funk of approaching controversy was in the air.

The Summer of '76

Two public health issues, swine flu and mammography guidelines, dominated the nation's attention during the summer of 1976. The first involved growing skepticism about a poorly conceived government plan to inoculate all Americans against a novel swine flu virus. This new virus had caused an outbreak at Fort Dix, New Jersey, in February of that year, sickening five hundred and causing one death. Fearing a repeat of the 1918–19 worldwide flu pandemic, the Ford administration immediately decided to begin development and testing of a vaccine against the virus—this even though there was no evidence of a developing epidemic in the months following the Fort Dix outbreak. The inoculation program eventually ended in disaster that fall after deaths and paralytic illnesses were linked to the vaccine.[31]

The second public health firestorm that summer was one that had been smoldering behind the scenes for several months. In September 1975 Dr. John C. Bailar III, NCI deputy associate director for cancer control, met with NCI director Dr. Frank Rauscher Jr. Bailar, a physician and biostatistician, had become increasingly concerned about the risk of radiation-induced breast cancer posed by BCDDP mammography, particularly to younger women. He had been making public statements about the issue for several months and had already presented the results of his analysis at the May 1975 meeting of the American Association for Cancer Research. To address Bailar's concerns, Rauscher appointed three expert committees to review the scientific underpinnings of the BCDDP. One of these, chaired by Dr. Arthur Upton, would study the issue of radiation risk.[32]

At this point the controversy was mainly taking place behind the scenes, an argument among researchers. There was very little public engagement on this issue. Yet the ACS felt that Bailar's assertions were a significant enough threat to the BCDDP that a joint press conference with the American College of Radiology was held in November 1975 to showcase positive early results from the program and to rebut Bailar's criticisms.[33] This incident illuminates two important dynamics in the evolution of screening mammography. First, early on, radiologists and the ACS created a formidable alliance in the advocacy and promotion of mammography. In fact, radiologists have always had a close relationship with the ACS. Six presidents of the ACS have been radiologists, including Dr. Justin Stein, whose term (1973–1974) coincided with the launch of the BCDDP.[34] This alliance has remained strong and has been a reliable bulwark through every crisis screening mammography has endured to this day. Second, these crises have frequently resulted in a standoff between the American College of Radiology and the ACS on the one hand and statisticians and epidemiologists on the other, passionate true believers versus dispassionate truth-seekers.

Bailar published "Mammography: A Contrary View" in the *Annals of Internal Medicine* in January 1976.[35] In it he detailed his analysis of the radiation hazards associated with screening mammography. He worked from what was known about breast cancer incidence rates in populations of women exposed to high doses of radiation, such as atomic bomb survivors, and extrapolated down to the lower doses associated with mammography. While Bailar was most concerned about the effects of radiation on younger women, whose breasts are more radiation sensitive, he ominously concluded, "Regretfully . . . there seems to be a possibility that the routine use of mammography in screening asymptomatic women may eventually take as many lives as it saves."[36] At around the same time, consumer activist Ralph Nader's Health Research Group uncovered documents showing that seventeen of the fifty-seven BCDDP mammography machines were producing radiation exposures in excess of program guidelines. The machine at the Georgetown University center in Washington, D.C., was delivering three times the maximum allowed radiation dose.[37]

These revelations and dire forebodings caused quite a stir. In March 1976 new BCDDP participant consent forms, for the first time describing the risks of radiation, were approved and quickly implemented.[38] These forms would be revised several more times that year, each time to expand on the issue of radiation risk. By the time the NCI convened a BCDDP project directors' meeting on July 15, 1976, to hear preliminary reports from the three expert panels, Bailar's warnings had already been widely disseminated in the lay press. By August the mounting public criticism of the BCDDP had government health officials on the defensive. New interim screening guidelines were hastily adopted by the NCI and ACS. The new guidelines reported that, on the basis of the work of Upton's panel, a single mammogram was believed to increase a woman's risk of breast cancer by 1 percent over her lifetime. Citing the benefits shown in the HIP study, the guidelines reaffirmed continued mammographic screening for women over fifty. Regarding younger women, however, the guidelines flatly stated, "We cannot recommend the routine use of mammography in screening asymptomatic women ages 35–49 years in the NCI/ACS BCDDP."[39]

If Betty Ford's and Happy Rockefeller's disclosures were the "action" of Newton's third law of motion, John Bailar's assertions were the "equal and opposite reaction." Almost immediately, enrollment at BCDDP sites saw a precipitous decline of up to 40 percent.[40] The possibility of mammography causing cancer prompted women of all ages to steer clear of the test. Not only were healthy women avoiding *screening* mammography, but also women with breast lumps who needed *diagnostic* mammography for evaluation of their symptoms were refusing the test.

Almost as soon as the new guidelines were published, it became clear that the ACS did not agree with this near-total prohibition on screening younger women. ACS officials resorted to an interesting tactic of simply defining womanhood between the ages of thirty-five and forty-nine as a risky state of being. Both its chief medical officer, Dr. Arthur Holleb, and its president, Dr. Benjamin Byrd Jr., were repeatedly quoted in lay publications making the dubious argument that up to 80 percent of women in that age group are in one or more high-risk categories and should be screened.[41] In a 1977 *Reader's Digest* interview, Byrd was asked, "How often should mammograms be done?" His response: "Mammograms should be done at the physician's discretion in women with a higher than normal risk of breast cancer. . . . In NCI-ACS experience, about 80% of women 35–50 meet one or another of these criteria."[42] Philip Strax, who ran one of the BCDDP sites in New York, promoted his own guidelines. Among his reasons for screening younger women was that "women who are worried about breast cancer . . . need [mammography] to prove they do not have the disease."[43]

Undeterred, the NCI tightened the restrictions further in May 1977, when it issued a modification of the interim guidelines. This modification allowed screening mammography in women aged thirty-five to forty-nine *only* if they had a personal history of breast cancer or had a mother or sister with the disease. Adherence to the new guidelines was made a contractual requirement for sites to continue participating in the BCDDP.[44]

The controversies surrounding the BCDDP led to the convening of the first National Institutes of Health (NIH) Consensus

Development Conference. Known officially as the NIH/NCI Consensus Development Meeting on Breast Cancer Screening, it was held September 14–16, 1977, and was open to the public. At this forum the final reports from the three expert committees established in October 1975 were presented. In addition, a fourth committee, chaired by Dr. Oliver Beahrs, presented results from a detailed review of the BCDDP. The Beahrs Report made several important recommendations. First, it recommended continuing the BCDDP as a demonstration project, as opposed to trying to convert it to a randomized controlled trial, as some had suggested. Second, it placed added restrictions on mammographic screening in women under fifty. Women between thirty-five and thirty-nine should undergo screening *only* if they had a *personal* history (not just a family history) of breast cancer. It reaffirmed the modified interim guidelines that allowed mammography screening for women forty to forty-nine who had a personal or a close family history of the disease. Third, it recommended that more randomized controlled trials, like the HIP, be conducted to find answers to questions that the BCDDP would never be able to answer. Questions such as the value of screening in women forty to forty-nine years of age and the optimum interval between screenings were highlighted.[45] The recommendations of the Beahrs Report were largely endorsed by the conference panelists. Significantly, the age-related mammography restrictions remained the official BCDDP policy through the remainder of the program.

Before concluding this chapter, I want briefly to consider one more public health issue that had its origin in the summer of 1976. This crisis, though, would not come to light until 1981. Epidemiologists with the U.S. Centers for Disease Control would later trace the earliest appearance of the AIDS virus in the United States to a small group of individuals, friends and lovers who, in the summer of 1976, were living in close proximity to one another in the West Village neighborhood of New York City.[46] The devastation wrought by this disease would give rise a decade later to the militant AIDS activism of the late 1980s, which in turn led to the rise of breast cancer activism in the early 1990s. This phenomenon was pivotal in the establishment of screening mammography in American culture and will be the subject of a later chapter.

(3)

THE AFTERMATH

Screening in the BCDDP was concluded in 1981, and the first results were published the following year.[1] Despite, or possibly because of, the controversy that had ensnared the program through much of its course, its sponsors proudly highlighted its accomplishments. Just over 280,000 participants had enrolled in the program, and about half (51.7 percent) completed all five screening rounds; 4,443 breast cancers were diagnosed. Of these, 3,557 diagnoses (80 percent) were directly attributable to screening (mammography or physical examination). The remaining 886 cases came to light either between annual screening visits or sometime after the participant completed the final round of screening. Of the 3,557 screening-detected cancers, 41 percent (1,481) were found on mammography alone. In the older HIP study, 33 percent of the screening-detected cancers were found on mammography alone. Among women fifty to fifty-nine years old, 41 percent of cancers in the HIP study and 42 percent in the BCDDP were detected by mammography alone. In women forty to forty-nine years old, 19.4 percent of cancers in the HIP were based on mammographic findings alone. In the BCDDP, this figure was nearly double, at 35.4 percent.

At surgery, 80 percent of BCDDP screening-detected cancers were found to have no involvement of lymph nodes, compared to 70 percent in the HIP.

Because the BCDDP was not designed as a scientific study, there was no control group of women who *did not* undergo screening. For that reason the BCDDP results could shed no light on the question of whether or not screening resulted in fewer breast cancer deaths (mortality reduction). Yet *mortality reduction* is the generally accepted standard by which the efficacy of a screening test is judged. If fewer screened than unscreened individuals die of the disease, the screening test can be declared effective.

These limitations notwithstanding, the ACS drew two critical conclusions from these early BCDDP data. The first was that the mammography of the 1970s was far superior to that of the 1960s. The rate of cancer detection in younger women, the percentage of cancers detected solely on mammography in women both over fifty and under fifty years old, and the rate of lymph node involvement were all significantly improved in the BCDDP versus the HIP. Second, it was therefore reasoned, since screening with the antiquated HIP mammography demonstrated a clear-cut mortality reduction for screened women over fifty, one could *assume* that such a mortality reduction would accrue to younger women as well with the use of modern mammography technology. The fact that the BCDDP's design could never positively prove this assumption did not hinder its acceptance.

The BCDDP's Legacy

In the history of mammography in the United States, the BCDDP was a seminal event. What the BCDDP *represented*, however, was as important as what it accomplished. As elegantly described by sociologist Maren Klawiter, the BCDDP represented a shift of the "mammographic gaze" into asymptomatic populations.[2] The shift began with the HIP but was accelerated with the BCDDP. Prior to this time, mammography was a diagnostic (as opposed to a screening) test, used to evaluate women with signs or symptoms of breast cancer. As the mammographic gaze became fixed on the population of women without symptoms, the message of early detection changed. The "Do Not Delay" message of much of the twentieth century became a "Go in Search" admonition.[3] This was a critical evolutionary development. The asymptomatic population is far larger than the population of women with symptoms. In becoming a test, essentially, for all women, screening mammography was guaranteed widespread dissemination and deep cultural assimilation. Had it remained a test used solely for women with symptoms, it would forever have been regarded like any other plain, unglamorous X-ray.

Another important consequence of the BCDDP was the rapid diffusion and adoption of a new breast cancer screening paradigm. As Klawiter notes, by the conclusion of the program, the concept "that perfectly healthy women exhibiting no signs of disease should be regularly screened with mammography" had become widely accepted by the public.[4] Screening mammography joined breast self-examination and clinical breast examination to form a new screening triumvirate that still stands today.[5]

The BCDDP resulted in a broadening of the definition of breast cancer. Prior to the advent of screening mammography, 98 to 99 percent of all breast cancers were what clinicians refer to as *invasive* (or *infiltrating*). This means that the breast cancer cells are not confined to the milk duct where the tumor originated but have invaded the tissue around the duct. Typically the tumor had grown to a sufficient size to form a lump that could be felt or demonstrate some other sign or symptom. Ductal carcinoma in situ (DCIS) is the stage in the development of a breast cancer when the cancer cells are still contained entirely within the milk duct. Usually there are no physical signs (such as a lump) at this point. For this reason, prior to the initiation of widespread screening mammography,

DCIS constituted 2 percent or less of all breast cancers.[6] Mammography happens to be uniquely suited to the diagnosis of DCIS. On a mammogram DCIS appears as small collections of calcium crystals (microcalcifications), which look like tiny white flecks on the X-ray. In the BCDDP, 11.5 percent of all cancers found in program participants were DCIS.[7] As screening mammography became more established in the medical culture, there was a 700 percent increase in its incidence between 1983 and 1998.[8] Today, DCIS constitutes approximately 20 to 25 percent of all newly diagnosed breast cancer cases. Up to 85 percent of all DCIS cases diagnosed today are found as a result of an abnormal mammogram.[9]

This explosion in the number of DCIS cases has been both a *cause* and an *effect* of screening mammography's success. Rapidly increasing DCIS diagnoses swelled the ranks of women diagnosed with breast cancer. This in turn helped elevate breast cancer to epidemic status—an epidemic for which more mammographic screening was presented as the cure. DCIS, however, is a poorly understood, unpredictable entity. It is believed that a large proportion (up to half) of these cases, if left alone, would not progress to the more dangerous invasive carcinoma.[10] DCIS that never progresses to invasive cancer is nonlethal. Thus, many DCIS cases actually represent what has been termed "overdiagnosis." This refers to the identification, through screening, of disease that, absent screening, would not have come to light in the patient's lifetime.[11] It is one of the harms or risks of screening. The difficulty is that there is currently no method to predict accurately which DCIS cases will progress and which ones will not. For that reason, essentially all women diagnosed with DCIS, approximately 53,000 in 2009,[12] undergo treatment, typically lumpectomy and radiation therapy, but also mastectomy in many cases.

The BCDDP spurred major improvements in mammographic quality. The dissemination of dedicated mammography machines as well as innovations in specialty film technology both occurred at an accelerated pace during the 1980s. These advancements drove down the radiation dose to approximately 10 percent of BCDDP levels and markedly improved overall image quality.

The final important effect of the BCDDP stems from the decision to perform a demonstration project rather than a clinical trial. As a demonstration project, the BCDDP was immensely successful in disseminating and establishing a culture of mammographic screening. One can only speculate how different the history of screening mammography would have been if instead the American Cancer Society and the National Cancer Institute had decided to sponsor a large research trial, with a control group, to determine if mammography was actually effective in women under fifty. The HIP trial had demonstrated benefit for women fifty to fifty-nine but had included an insufficient number of younger women to answer the question definitively for that age group. By simply assuming benefit where none had been proven and forging ahead with a demonstration program, BCDDP sponsors sowed the seeds of the controversy that erupted in the summer of 1976. This controversy about the benefits of mammography in women under fifty remains unsettled to this day.

The Mainstreaming of Mammography

With the end of the BCDDP era, the mammographic gaze was about to become unblinkingly riveted on the population of healthy women. This would be accomplished through the adoption and aggressive promotion of screening guidelines by prominent organizations. At this point in its history, screening mammography had two powerful and passionate allies: the ACS and the American College of Radiology (ACR). Apart from the subsequent emergence of the breast cancer activist movement, which I consider later, there has been no more consequential alliance in the establishment of the culture of mammographic screening.

In 1983 the ACS freed itself from the constraints of its 1977 agreement with the National Cancer Institute regarding screening in younger women. Citing the early BCDDP results, it published new breast cancer screening guidelines that recommended mammography every one to two years for women forty to forty-nine and annual mammography for women over fifty.[13] This immediately added 12 million women to the 34 million women over fifty for whom routine screening was recommended. While not openly criticizing this action, the NCI stated that it would not follow suit. It would maintain its 1977 stance, which recommended screening for women in their forties only if they were at high risk.[14] Thus the fault line between the ACS and the NCI that had first become evident in 1976–77 had now fully ruptured. The two would reconcile later in the decade but would continue to have a conflicted relationship through much of the subsequent history of screening mammography.

The ACR, owing the NCI no deference, had long ago begun recommending screening for women in their forties. In 1976, at the height of the BCDDP controversy, it mounted a vigorous defense of mammographic screening and adopted a position that women forty to forty-nine years old should be screened every one to three years.[15] At the time, it offered no scientific justification for this recommendation. There was none. In fact, in its 1976 announcement the ACR conceded as much, noting, "Since there is now no definite scientific evidence with regard to: 1) optimal age for the initial mammogram; 2) frequency of examination; 3) data on possible long term radiation risk; this statement is being issued as a summary of current *informed opinion*." The ACR statement further highlighted the lack of a scientific basis for the recommendation by invoking the "promise" of mammography: "Mammography at appropriate intervals in asymptomatic women over age 35 promises to reduce significantly the number of deaths from breast cancer."[16] In 1982, shortly after the publication of the early BCDDP results, the ACR broadened its guidelines to recommend screening for women in their forties every one to two years.[17]

As the 1980s drew to a close, there was a hodgepodge of screening guidelines published by various medical organizations. Wanting to present a unified message to the public, the ACR, under the leadership of Dr. Gerald Dodd, professor of radiology at the University of Texas M. D. Anderson Cancer Center (and a future ACS president), organized the National Medical Roundtable on Mammography. This group reviewed both the latest BCDDP survival results and a recently published reanalysis of HIP data which showed that ten to eighteen years after entering the study, HIP participants who were forty to forty-nine at enrollment had a statistically significant reduction in breast cancer mortality.[18] The methodology used in this new analysis was not universally accepted, and the conclusions were controversial.[19] This was, however, the first time such a benefit had been demonstrated for women under fifty, and it was the evidence the ACR and ACS needed in order to argue persuasively for more aggressive screening.

Eleven organizations, including the American Medical Association and the NCI, concurred when the Medical Roundtable published its consensus guidelines in July 1989.[20] These guidelines called for screening mammography every one to two years for women aged forty to forty-nine and annual mammography thereafter.[21]

Conspicuously absent from the list of screening supporters were the U.S. Preventive Services Task Force and the American College of Physicians. The Preventive Services Task Force was convened by the U.S. Public Health Service in 1984, charged with periodically reviewing the scientific evidence for or against a wide array of clinical preventive services, including cancer screening. Its recommendations are heavily relied on by government health policymakers and private industry. In its 1989 *Guide to Clinical Preventive Services*, the Task Force rejected screening mammography in women under fifty, citing concerns about costs and high rates of false positive results.[22]

The American College of Physicians, the largest medical specialty society (including general internists and internal medicine subspecialists), also demurred on the "consensus" guidelines. It chose, instead, to stand by its 1985 guidelines that discouraged screening women in their forties, except those at high risk.[23]

(4)

A TALE OF TWO EPIDEMICS

*I am sick of everyone in this community who tells me to
stop creating a panic. How many of us have to die before
you get scared off your ass and into action?*

LARRY KRAMER, playwright and AIDS activist, 1983

*If we told the men in this country that one in nine were
going to lose a testicle, they'd think it was an epidemic
and do something about it.*

ELENORE PRED, breast cancer activist, 1991

In June 1981 the U.S. Centers for Disease Control (CDC) published a brief report on five previously healthy gay men in Los Angeles who had been diagnosed with a rare form of pneumonia. Two of them had died.[1] At the time, no one could have anticipated the public health cataclysm that was about to be unleashed upon the world. During the first two years of what would become known as the AIDS epidemic, cases increased exponentially. By September 1982, 593 cases had been reported, and 243 patients (41 percent) had died.[2] One year later the CDC reported 2,259 cases and 917 deaths. Of these 2,259 cases, 58 (3 percent) had been diagnosed prior to 1981, 231 (10 percent) in 1981, 883 (39 percent) in 1982, and 1,087 (48 percent) during the period from January through September 1983.[3]

Given the fury with which this new and devastatingly efficient killer appeared on the scene, it was greeted with remarkable indifference. AIDS had emerged during the first few months of Ronald Reagan's presidency. Reagan had been elected by campaigning on a platform of social and fiscal conservatism. Once in office, he enacted massive cuts in nonmilitary government expenditures. In particular, the CDC's budget was slashed in half. For the first several years of the AIDS epidemic, the CDC and the National Institutes of Health received minuscule resources to deal with it. As noted by investigative journalist Randy Shilts in *And the Band Played On*, "people died while Reagan administration officials ignored pleas from government scientists and did not allocate adequate funding for AIDS research until the epidemic had already spread throughout the country."[4] Reagan himself made no public comments on the AIDS epidemic until May 1987, halfway through his second presidential term, a full six years after the devastation began.[5]

Government officials were not the only ones suffering from AIDS-related indifference. Up until 1985 the media largely ignored the crisis. In those early years of the epidemic, the new "gay disease" was considered irrelevant and discussion of gay sexual practices unacceptable to a "mainstream" American audience.[6] Even though cases of AIDS had begun to be observed among heterosexuals, including male intravenous drug abusers and their female sexual partners, Haitian immigrants, hemophiliacs, and infants born to women with the illness, AIDS was still largely a disease of socially marginalized individuals. Even the gay press was, early on, ambivalent about AIDS. Shame and finger-pointing (often directed at those gays who lived a "fast-lane" lifestyle) were pervasive in articles from that period.[7]

AIDS Activism

By the time AIDS came along, the radical activism of the gay liberation movement of the 1960s and 1970s had long since faded. The gay community of the 1980s was fast becoming a traditional interest group, more concerned with political organizing and working inside the system, as opposed to militant activism.[8] Expressions of gay pride in the 1960s and 1970s tended to highlight and celebrate gay sexual difference. By the early to mid-1980s, gay pride frequently pointed instead to similarities with the dominant society.[9]

Given this evolution in the conception of gay pride, the gay community's response in the early years of the AIDS epidemic was socially conforming. The goals of this early activism were twofold: providing care and support to the exploding numbers of sick and dying, and raising funds for research.[10] Service organizations such as the New York Gay Men's Health Crisis, founded in 1981, developed in many urban gay centers. The Gay Men's Health Crisis achieved moderate fund-raising success, but it soon became clear that it would never be able to meet the challenges of this epidemic. With corporate donations almost nonexistent and government funding miserly, there simply wasn't enough money in the gay community to fund the anti-AIDS effort adequately. AIDS activists longed for an American Cancer Society–like organization that would educate gays and demand more government research funds.[11]

As early as 1983 some leaders in the gay and lesbian community, notably Larry Kramer of the Gay Men's Health Crisis and Virginia Apuzzo of the National Gay Task Force, had begun advocating a return to the militant activism of the 1960s as the only way to spur government and society to action.[12] These early calls for the community to take to the streets went largely unheeded, however. In fact, social scientist Dennis Altman, writing in the mid-1980s, observed, "Perhaps the greatest gap in AIDS politicking is the lack of a genuine mass mobilization behind demands for a greater government response to AIDS."[13]

In June 1986 the U.S. Supreme Court handed down a 5–4 ruling that upheld the state of Georgia's anti-sodomy statute in the case of *Bowers v. Hardwick*. In it the Court asserted that the rights of privacy and liberty did not extend to acts of homosexual sodomy in a private home between consenting adults.[14]

The *Hardwick* decision had an immediate and galvanizing effect on the gay and lesbian community. By this time there had been 28,000 diagnosed AIDS cases and nearly 16,000 deaths.[15] *Hardwick* was seen as an unqualified rejection of homosexuality by straight America and brought into sharp focus the horrific effects of all those years of neglect by government and society.

Almost immediately AIDS activism, which had previously been service and support oriented, took on a tone of strident militancy. Street protests, demonstrations, sit-ins, and other acts of civil disobedience broke out in cities all over the country and continued for months. Anger that had been suppressed for years erupted forcefully and uncontrollably. Confrontational direct-action AIDS groups, most notably the Silence = Death Project, the Lavender Hill Mob, and the AIDS Coalition to Unleash Power (ACT UP), formed in the immediate aftermath of *Hardwick*.[16] These groups took particular aim at the U.S. Food and Drug Administration (FDA), which some activists renamed the "Federal Death Administration" for its slow approval of drugs that had shown promise in phase 1 trials, and at the drug company Burroughs Wellcome over the high cost of AZT, the only AIDS drug available at the time.[17] In fact the primary goal of this new activism was to bring new therapies more rapidly to the suffering and dying. "Drugs into bodies" became ACT UP's rallying cry. The new post-*Hardwick* AIDS activism reached a peak on October 11, 1987, when hundreds of thousands of activists converged on Washington, D.C. The crowd included AIDS patients, some in wheelchairs, gays, lesbians, and heterosexual supporters of gay rights. They marched past the Reagan White House and gathered on the National Mall for an afternoon rally. The focal point of the rally was a giant quilt, memorializing the 25,000 individuals who had died of the disease.[18]

In the late 1980s AIDS activism scored important victories on both the legislative and the scientific fronts. In October 1988 Congress passed a comprehensive $1 billion AIDS bill, which represented the first stand-alone AIDS funding legislation since the start of the epidemic. It included $600 million in research funding as well as a mandate that the Public Health Service hire an additional 780 full-time employees to work on AIDS research. Funds for educational programs, home health care, and voluntary testing were also included in the new law.[19]

Activists forced changes at the FDA that significantly shortened the drug approval process.[20] They also forced changes at the National Institute of Allergy and Immunology (part of the National Institutes of Health) to increase significantly the representation of women and ethnic minorities in federally funded research trials. And they forced changes in the methodology of those trials so that enrolled research subjects were allowed simultaneously to take medications to treat the complications of AIDS, something they had previously been prohibited from doing. Finally, activists gained the respect of the research establishment and were granted a seat at the table on NIH and FDA advisory committees and other private and public research panels. In this way they were able to have a direct effect on decisions about the direction of AIDS research.[21]

One in Ten (. . . Nine . . . Eight . . .)

Meanwhile, after the acrimony that characterized the conclusion of the BCDDP, mammography resided in the shadows for much of the 1980s. In the early part of the decade, what little was written about breast cancer screening in the popular press focused largely on alternatives to mammography. These were frequently presented as safer options, as they did not involve harmful radiation. Breast self-examination, the new technology of ultrasound, and a light scanning technique known as transillumination were widely written about.[22]

The period from 1987 through 1992 saw the emergence of the modern breast cancer activist movement. Though it began slowly, it quickly gained steam and became a formidable social and political force in a very short space of time. The story of breast cancer activism in these years has received extensive treatment in scholarly and popular publications, and the lessons of this period are many. One lesson, however, is inescapable: the story of this modern period of breast cancer activism is an important chapter in *mammography*'s story. It tells how mammography became fully assimilated in American culture. It tells how the mantra of early detection finally gained widespread acceptance. It tells how mammography was launched on a trajectory that would eventually make it the second most commonly performed cancer screening test and how, in the process, a multibillion-dollar industry grew up around it.

At this point in its history, for mammographic screening to achieve widespread acceptance, there were three necessary conditions: doctors would have to recommend it, government and private insurance would have to cover it, and women would have to feel an urgent need for it. As we saw in the last chapter, the American Cancer Society's principal ally in its mammography campaign, the American College of Radiology, convened a summit of eleven medical organizations in 1989 and achieved a consensus on guidelines promoting screening in women starting at age forty. As a result of this and other efforts, by 1989, 96 percent of physicians surveyed reported recommending screening mammography to their patients. The same survey performed in 1984 had found only 49 percent of physicians recommending screening.[23]

The epidemic narrative that developed around breast cancer in the late 1980s would serve as a highly effective focusing event. It would drive home to the masses of healthy American women the urgency of the breast cancer problem and the need for regular screening. This increased awareness and anxiety would, in turn, force lawmakers to enact legislation promoting mammography and breast cancer research.

In October 1987 President Ronald Reagan announced that his wife, Nancy, had been successfully treated for breast cancer. Nancy Reagan's diagnosis differed from Betty Ford's and Happy Rockefeller's in one important regard: while Mrs. Ford and Mrs. Rockefeller had both had tumors that were found on physical examination, Nancy Reagan had a 7 mm (about the size of a lemon seed) ductal carcinoma in situ, picked up on a routine *screening* mammogram.[24] This mammographic "save" involving the first lady predictably received widespread attention in the press and among the public at large. Its impact was swiftly felt at mammography centers across the country. Phones were reported to be "ringing off the hook," and patient volumes doubled at many facilities.[25]

This episode by itself might have been a blip in the use of mammography, as had been the case with the Ford-Rockefeller incident thirteen years earlier, were it not for one fact. In the late 1980s, epidemic anxiety was palpable and widespread. The public was paying attention to the growing AIDS crisis. The images of AIDS activists demanding government action were everywhere.

In 1985 the American Cancer Society announced that the lifetime probability of an American Caucasian woman developing breast cancer had risen from one in thirteen to one in ten over the past decade.[26] In fact the 1978 incidence of breast cancer was 84 cases per 100,000 population. By 1987 it had increased by 35 percent to 113 cases per 100,000. In 1978 there were 90,000 new cases and 34,000 deaths. In 1987 there were 130,000 new cases and 41,000 deaths. These facts, though widely known, received little attention prior to Nancy Reagan's diagnosis.

Following Mrs. Reagan's encounter with breast cancer, the popular press began to fill with articles highlighting the rapidly rising breast cancer rates. These articles typically had a foreboding tone, describing a baffling, out-of-control disease, not unlike AIDS. By the time the ACS announced, in January 1991, that the lifetime probability of a woman's developing breast cancer had increased to one in nine, the idea that the nation was experiencing an all-out breast cancer epidemic had fully taken hold. Sensational headlines such as "Every Thirteen Minutes, Another Woman Dies of Breast Cancer" in the *Ladies' Home Journal* and "The Breast Cancer Epidemic: Women Aren't Just Scared, We're Mad" in *McCall's* were typical of this period.[27]

Breast cancer survivors took note of the successes of militant AIDS activism and started forming their own organizations. Whereas the women's health movement of the late 1960s and 1970s was characterized by self-help and support, the modern breast cancer activist movement adopted the direct political action model of AIDS activists. In fact, many women were active in both movements simultaneously. Elenore Pred, who founded the group Breast Cancer Action, was reported in a 1990 *Newsweek* article to have spoken to the editors of *AIDS Treatment News* and received a crash course in their techniques prior to forming her organization. "I learned to question the decisions of the AMA, the FDA and the American Cancer Society," she was reported to have said.[28] On Mother's Day in 1991, one thousand Breast Cancer Action activists and others marched on the California state capitol in Sacramento, demanding more breast cancer funding.[29] "We are very angry . . . and we must stop treating this disease as a personal tragedy" was her frequent rallying cry.[30]

It wasn't long, however, before tensions arose between the two activist communities. In 1990, U.S. government research expenditures were $1.1 billion for AIDS and $77 million for breast cancer.[31] Breast cancer activists like the noted breast surgeon Susan Love publicly condemned this funding discrepancy, given that breast cancer had claimed six times as many lives in the past decade as had AIDS.[32]

The goals of the modern breast cancer activist movement were, broadly speaking, increased research funding, both to find a cure and to discover the environmental causes of breast cancer, and also wider insurance coverage for screening mammography. In a 1990 survey by the Jacobs Institute of Women's Health, 65 percent of white women and 58 percent of African American women over the age of forty reported having had at least one screening mammogram. The corresponding figures for 1987 were 39 and 30 percent, respectively. In 1990, 31 percent reported having had mammograms according to the 1989 guidelines of the American Cancer Society.[33] Those guidelines called for mammography every one to two years for women aged forty to forty-nine and annually thereafter. Of those women who had never had a mammogram, fear of radiation and the high cost were cited as major barriers. At that time a screening mammogram cost between $50 and $150. Including the interpretation fee, the total cost could run as high as $200. In the same 1990 survey, 45 percent of respondents stated that they would be unwilling to pay $150 for a screening mammogram.

The dramatic increase in screening mammography rates between 1987 and 1990 did not occur simply because American women had begun to heed the advice of the ACS. Cost was clearly an impediment that would have to be overcome. This issue was attacked on two fronts: at state capitols and in Washington, D.C. Local ACS chapters and other breast cancer activist groups pressured state legislatures all across the country to enact legislation requiring insurance companies to cover screening mammography or to provide such coverage as an optional benefit. It should be noted that up until this time, it was virtually unheard of for third-party payers to cover preventive services. In 1986, significantly aided by the untiring efforts of breast cancer patient-activist Rose Kushner, Maryland became the first state to enact such legislation.[34] In 1987 the Susan G. Komen Breast Cancer Foundation, a breast cancer advocacy organization formed in 1982, pressured Texas state lawmakers and secured insurance coverage for screening mammography.[35] California and Massachusetts also passed similar laws that year. By 1990, thirty-three states and by 1992, forty-two states and the District of Columbia had enacted laws promoting insurance coverage for screening mammography.[36]

In the U.S. Congress, Representative Mary Rose Oakar, an Ohio Democrat whose sister had been diagnosed with breast cancer, had been trying unsuccessfully since 1983 to find a Senate co-sponsor for a bill to mandate Medicare coverage for screening mammography. With pressure from Rose Kushner and a letter-writing campaign by members of the National Alliance of Breast Cancer Organizations, mammography coverage was added to the Medicare Catastrophic Coverage Act of 1988.[37] The new law provided coverage for screening mammography for women beginning at age forty. This victory was short-lived, however. Large numbers of Medicare recipients loudly protested a new surtax that legislators had included in the law as a means of funding its enhanced benefits. Under pressure, Congress repealed the law in 1989.[38] The mammography provisions, however, reemerged as part of the 1990 Omnibus Budget Reconciliation Act, and Medicare coverage for screening mammography began in January 1991. At around the same time, the Breast and Cervical Cancer Mortality Prevention Act of 1990 provided federal grants ($64 million awarded in the first year) to state health agencies to make Pap smears and screening mammography available to low-income women.[39]

It was also around this time that breast cancer activists scored one of their most remarkable legislative victories. The National Breast Cancer Coalition was founded in 1991, the year the ACS began publicizing the new one-in-nine lifetime risk figure for breast cancer. Its first president, Fran Visco, set out on an ambitious program to collect 175,000 letters from supporters, one for each of the projected new breast cancer cases that year. The campaign succeeded beyond expectations. Over 600,000 letters were collected and delivered to Congress and the Bush White House in the fall of 1991.[40] These letters demanded more funding for breast cancer research. Senator Tom Harkin, an Iowa Democrat who had lost two sisters to breast cancer, chaired the Senate committee overseeing NIH funding. Growth in nonmilitary government spending was at the time severely restricted under the Budget Enforcement Act of 1990. Through some fancy legislative footwork, Harkin orchestrated the appropriation of $400 million of new funding for breast cancer research, $210 million of which was placed in the budget of the Department of Defense.

In October 1991 the nation was engrossed by the televised drama unfolding in a U.S. Senate hearing room, where President George H. W. Bush's nomination of Judge Clarence Thomas to the U.S. Supreme Court was being considered. Judge Thomas was publicly accused of sexual harassment by Anita F. Hill, a law professor at the University of Oklahoma. The alleged harassment had occurred years earlier, when Thomas was directing the Office of Civil Rights in the Department of Education and Hill was his assistant.[41] The hearings became a riveting "he said/she said" drama filled with subtexts of race, sex, and power. In the end, it was widely felt that Hill's allegations were not taken seriously and that she was treated poorly by the all-male Senate Judiciary Committee.

The Thomas hearings helped to usher in the "Year of the Woman," as the 1992 federal election cycle was dubbed. Women made significant gains in the U.S. Congress, increasing their representation in the House of Representative from twenty-eight to forty-seven and in the Senate from three to six.[42] This, along with the election of a Democratic president, William J. Clinton, provided an environment in which women's health became a potent issue for legislators attempting to win favor with female constituents.[43]

As I conclude this section I must consider one additional major piece of mammography legislation that emerged during this period of activism. In the 1980s there was an explosion in the number of mammography facilities in the United States. There were fewer than two hundred such facilities in 1982 but 3,939 in 1985, 6,404 in

1988, and approximately 10,000 by 1992.[44] As early as 1985, however, it was clear that in many cases, this increased quantity did not translate to improved quality. In a nationwide survey of mammography facilities in 1985, the Food and Drug Administration found that at 36 percent of them, the quality of the mammographic images was unacceptable. Furthermore, even though dedicated mammography machines had been widely available since the early 1970s, 15 percent of surveyed facilities were still using general purpose X-ray equipment for mammography.[45] Largely on the basis of these findings, the American College of Radiology, with a grant from the American Cancer Society, initiated a voluntary accreditation program for mammography facilities in August 1987. As this was a voluntary program, participation rates were low for the first several years. By March 1988, 967 facilities and by May 1990, 2,436 facilities had applied for accreditation. Approximately 30 percent of applicants failed on the first attempt, the vast majority because of poor image quality.[46]

Not only were there significant issues with the technical quality of the mammography films being produced at facilities around the country, but also there were growing concerns about the radiologists who were interpreting them. In June 1990, *NBC Nightly News* investigative correspondent Michele Gillen presented a three-part series on the problem of poor-quality mammography. She highlighted several tragic cases of misread mammograms. These were women who had been falsely reassured that they were cancer free, only to find out later, sometimes much later, that their mammograms had been misinterpreted and they now had advanced breast cancer.[47]

Even though the new Medicare mammography coverage legislation that took effect in January 1991 included some quality standards for participating facilities, and even though some states had begun setting their own standards, it was clear that a uniform set of national standards would be needed to address properly the demonstrated inconsistencies in mammography quality. Congress passed the Mammography Quality Standards Act in 1992. This new law gave the FDA sweeping authority to regulate mammography throughout the United States. Facilities were required to be accredited and undergo an annual on-site FDA inspection. The law's provisions governed the technical aspects of mammography (dedicated machines were now required), and the qualifications of the technologists who performed and the radiologists who interpreted the studies. The new law also required, for the first time, that patients receive a written summary of their mammography results directly from the facility.

Fear as a Motivator

The physical diffusion and cultural assimilation of screening mammography were significantly aided by the epidemic narrative that grew up around breast cancer in the late 1980s. The dominant message of the time, largely developed and advanced by the ACS but also promoted by the National Cancer Institute and the media, was that breast cancer rates were rising rapidly; it was now striking one in ten (. . . nine . . . eight) American women; breast cancer is 90–100 percent curable if caught early; and mammography is the best way to catch it early. This message appeared in print, television news programs, and public service announcements. 1 in 9: The Long Island Breast Cancer Action Coalition even placed the central tenet right in its organization's name. It was a simple, neatly packaged message, laying out the problem and giving the solution in fifteen seconds or less. In its simplicity, however, many important facts were overlooked or ignored.

One of the important facts missing from this pervasive admonition was that screening mammography itself was largely responsible for the breast cancer "epidemic." The rise in breast cancer cases was not a true epidemic but rather a predictable statistical phenomenon. For as long as records have been maintained, the breast cancer incidence rate has increased by approximately 1 percent per year. The dramatic increase in incidence above this 1 percent per year background trend observed in the late 1980s to early 1990s was completely explained, first, by increased screening, finding cases in the present that would otherwise have come to light sometime in the future (accounting for 87 percent of the increase), and second, by the fact that women were living longer; that is, fewer women were dying early of other causes, thereby increasing the number of women who could possibly contract breast cancer (accounting for 13 percent of the increase).[48]

Also missing was any context or explanation of the one in ten (. . . nine . . . eight) statistic. The fact that it represents a lifetime probability of developing breast cancer sometime between birth and age 110 or that the likelihood of developing breast cancer at any specific age is significantly lower than one in ten (. . . nine . . . eight) was rarely presented to the public. On the contrary, the ACS readily admitted promoting this largely meaningless statistic primarily for its shock value. Its purpose was to drive mammography screening through fear. In a March 1992 *New York Times* article, ACS spokesperson JoAnn Schellenback conceded: "The 1-in-9 is meant to be a jolt. We use it to remind people that the problem hasn't gone away. It's meant to be more of a metaphor more than a hard figure. Many younger women look at nine of their friends and think 'One of us is going to get cancer *this year*." The truth is that one of them will get cancer in their lifetime—but probably not until she's over 65."[49] Perfectly rational, healthy women began to view their breasts as ticking time bombs. This relentless messaging has resulted in a pervasive tendency for healthy women to overestimate both their own personal risk of breast cancer and the potential benefits of mammography.[50] In this way, the establishment of a culture of mammographic screening was greatly aided.

(5)

AGE IS NOTHING BUT A NUMBER

It has been frequently observed that the United States is virtually alone among developed countries in its support for screening mammography in women under fifty. This support has wavered little since the technology was introduced. This apparent American consensus on screening, however, is only an illusion. Just beneath the veneer of unanimity lies a dispute that will not die. Since 1976, every time mammography has become embroiled in controversy, the question of screening women in their forties has been the central issue. In the 1970s this issue nearly aborted mammography's debut during the Breast Cancer Detection Demonstration Project, and in the 1990s the same controversy arose twice, almost bringing the ascendancy of mammography to a complete halt.

Empowering Women to Decide for Themselves

The first sensational sentence of an article in the *Sunday Times* of London on June 2, 1991, was enough to panic even the most dispassionate professional. It read, "Middle-aged women who have regular mammograms are more likely to die from breast cancer than women who are not screened, according to dramatic new research."[1] The article went on to detail results from a major mammography screening trial performed in Canada. Even though the official results were not yet published (and would not be for over a year), study data were leaked to the press and had begun to circulate.

The Canadian National Breast Screening Study: 1 (CNBSS-1, or Canadian Trial), sponsored by the National Cancer Institute of Canada, was the first study specifically designed to determine whether or not screening mammography is effective in women under fifty. It utilized the scientifically favored randomized controlled trial methodology. Starting in 1980, researchers eventually recruited fifty thousand healthy women aged forty to forty-nine and randomly assigned them to one of two groups. The MP group received mammography and physical examination of the breasts annually, and the UC (usual care) group had one initial physical examination of the breasts but no subsequent examinations and no mammography. The trial was conducted for four years, and participants were followed for an average of eight years.

Even though leaked preliminary results had been appearing in the lay press for over a year, when the official results were published in November 1992, mammography was dragged into a whirlpool of controversy. The results of the Canadian Trial showed that after eight years of follow-up, routine mammography did not reduce the death rate from breast cancer among women forty to forty-nine.[2] In fact there were 36 percent *more* (thirty-eight as opposed to twenty-eight) breast cancer deaths in the MP group than in the UC group.[3] The difference was not statistically significant, meaning that it could have been caused simply by chance. Nevertheless, the idea that screening could *possibly* be harmful was alarming.

Almost immediately, the Canadian Trial came under a barrage of withering criticism. In lay and professional publications, the backers of screening for women under fifty, led by the American Cancer Society and the American College of Radiology, denounced the study as so deeply flawed that its results were untrustworthy and should be ignored. Critics deplored what they viewed as faulty methodology used for assigning participants to the two study groups, an inadequate number of participants, and the limited length of follow-up. But they reserved their harshest criticism for the quality of the CNBSS mammograms, pointing to the fact that two prominent U.S. radiologists who had served as outside consultants had resigned in protest over this issue. In its official statement on the Canadian Trial, the ACR concluded dismissively, "Perhaps the most important result of the [C]NBSS is the demonstration that poor mammography . . . reduces the effectiveness of screening."[4]

Shortly after the publication of the CNBSS-1 results, both the ACS and the NCI announced plans to convene separate scientific conferences to review the latest data on screening mammography, especially in women under fifty. At this point the state of the science was essentially the following. There had been eight major trials of the effectiveness of screening mammography that included women in the forty to forty-nine age group. These were randomized controlled trials, in which participants were assigned at random to "screening" or "no screening" groups. Even though all eight trials included women under fifty, only the CNBSS-1 was *specifically designed* to study this age demographic. Of these eight studies, none showed a statistically significant[5] reduction in mortality within the first ten years of initiating screening. One, the HIP study, showed a possible reduction in mortality after ten to eighteen years. In contrast, all studies save one showed a statistically significant reduction in mortality for screened women over the age of fifty. In addition to those studies, the BCDDP, though not designed as a scientific trial, showed that real-world mammography in the 1970s was equally effective in finding early stage breast cancer in women under fifty as in women over fifty.

The American Cancer Society's Workshop on Breast Cancer Detection in Younger Women was held February 1–2, 1993. The first day was devoted to a review of the available data. At least five of the six speakers who were selected for this task were known, on the basis of prior written and oral comments, to favor screening in women under fifty.[6] Even though Dr. Cornelia Baines, deputy director of the Canadian Trial, was invited to the conference, program organizers chose not to ask her to make a formal presentation on the study. Instead, Curtis Mettlin, an epidemiologist who chaired the ACS's Committee on Cancer Prevention and Detection, presented a bruising critique of the CNBSS-1.[7] The radiologists Daniel Kopans of Massachusetts General Hospital and Lazlo Tabar of Central Hospital in Falun, Sweden, also harshly panned the Canadian study during their presentations. Baines was relegated to the lesser role of panel discussion participant, from which position she valiantly tried to rebut the critics. Unsurprisingly, at the conclusion of its two-day conference, the ACS publicly reaffirmed its stance that women under fifty should undergo routine screening.

The National Cancer Institute's International Workshop on Screening for Breast Cancer was held on February 24–25, 1993. It was chaired by Dr. Suzanne Fletcher, who had previously stated her opposition to screening women under fifty. In a December 1992 article commenting on the renewed under-fifty screening controversy, Fletcher opined: "Medical scientists and physicians do not do modern women a service by promulgating a screening practice that medical science has not been able to substantiate after so many tries. We serve them far better by continuing the search for a practice that does work."[8] After reviewing essentially the same scientific data that the ACS had reviewed a mere three weeks earlier, the NCI concluded that there was no proof that screening mammography in women aged forty to forty-nine saves lives.[9] It nevertheless stopped short of reversing its 1989 guidelines advocating screening every one to two years for this group of women. This restraint would not last long.

That two respected cancer organizations could arrive at diametrically opposed conclusions from a review of the same data set is not as surprising as it may seem. The situation represented a classic "glass half full/glass half empty" paradox. On the one hand, groups such as the American Cancer Society and the American College of Radiology argued that since there was no scientific proof that screening in women under fifty was actually *harmful,* and since there was an abundance of evidence that screening was highly effective in women over fifty, screening younger women should be *presumed* effective. In other words, public policy should give screening for younger women the benefit of the doubt. In fact, Daniel Kopans, who achieved national prominence during this period as one of the most passionate apologists for early screening, repeatedly contended that there was nothing "magical" about the age of fifty.[10] There was no dramatic biological change that took place the moment a woman completed five decades of life. Furthermore, both the ACR and ACS repeatedly made the argument that none of the research trials completed thus far had been properly designed or executed to answer the question accurately. They estimated that in order to prove the effectiveness of screening mammography in women under fifty, a study would need to recruit 500,000 participants. Yet all the published studies combined included fewer than 170,000 women aged forty to forty-nine.[11] In the absence of reliable data, they reasoned, it would be unwise and dangerous to reverse course on the now decade-long public health effort to promote mammography as a life-saving test for all women over forty.

On the other hand, groups such as the NCI and the U.S. Preventive Services Task Force took the approach that if screening had not been *proven* effective, it must be considered *ineffective.* This position was aptly stated by Barbara K. Rimer, Ph.D., then of the Duke University Comprehensive Cancer Center. "Giving younger women false hope about the value of mammography is a disservice," she argued. "The National Cancer Institute owes it to women to tell them the truth. . . . In public health advice, we need a great deal of certainty, and there is no scientific support for a public health policy that advocates routine screening in this age group."[12]

In October 1993 the Board of Scientific Counselors, an NCI advisory board, recommended that, given the outcome of the February conference, the NCI should immediately rescind its guideline for routine mammography in women under fifty and replace it with a statement of the current evidence so that women could make up their own minds.[13] The recommendation was passed on to another NCI advisory body, the National Cancer Advisory Board. By a 14–1 vote, it approved a motion advising that, despite the controversy, the NCI should *defer* making any changes to its current guidelines supporting screening under age fifty.[14]

The new political environment in Washington, D.C., following the 1992 "Year of the Woman" national elections made it inevitable that this mammography dispute would become infused with a heavy dose of politics. In September 1993 the new president, Bill Clinton, presented to Congress and the nation his administration's vision for reforming the U.S. health care system. The Health Security Act was the latest federal attempt at providing all Americans with health care coverage. The comprehensive benefits package included in the Clinton plan provided for mammography screening every one to two years, starting at age fifty. It did not include a mandate for screening women under fifty. Thus it was inescapable when the NCI, in December 1993, formally dropped its guideline for screening women under fifty, replacing it with a statement of evidence as the Board of Scientific Counselors had advised, that critics would cry politics. Dr. Bernadine Healy, former director of the National Institutes of Health under President George H. W. Bush, accused the Clinton administration of "using the NCI's new position to justify a cost-based decision to limit women's health care choices—to limit their access to mammography at a time when breast cancer is reaching epidemic proportions."[15]

In the U.S. House of Representatives, twenty-nine lawmakers signed on to a "Sense of the House" resolution put forth by Representative Edolphus Towns, a Democrat from New York, urging that any comprehensive benefits package approved under health care reform include coverage for mammography screening of women forty to forty-nine.[16] Furthermore, the Human Resources and Intergovernmental Relations Subcommittee, chaired by Representative Towns, launched an aggressive investigation into the NCI's actions leading up to the controversial mammography decision. As part of its investigation, the subcommittee held a hearing on the matter on March 8, 1994. Dr. Samuel Broder, NCI director, was ordered to appear and answer members' questions. During the hearing Broder endured sharp questioning in which the subcommittee first dissected, then denounced, the process that the NCI had followed in its yearlong deliberations. In addition to Broder, eight other witnesses were invited to speak at the hearing. These were surgeons, radiologists, a representative of the ACS, and the mother of a young woman who had died of breast cancer at twenty-two. All were passionately opposed to the NCI's actions. No witnesses supportive of the NCI's position had been invited to address the subcommittee.[17] In its report *Misused Science: The National Cancer Institute's Elimination of Mammography Guidelines for Women in Their Forties*, Towns's subcommittee was harshly critical of the NCI and Director Broder.[18] The report blasted the NCI for considering only data from randomized controlled trials in its February 1993 International Workshop, for excluding nontrial data supportive of mammography (such as the BCDDP), for "stacking" the panel with opponents of under-fifty screening so that the results were a foregone conclusion, and for causing mass confusion among the American public about the value of mammography. In sum, the NCI's entire February 1993 exercise was denounced as "flawed from the start" and a waste of "many taxpayer dollars."[19]

Do Over

In the end, the government and public pressure were insufficient to cause the NCI to reverse itself. Its new screening guidelines would stand for several years. The whole episode and its aftermath would later be described by Republican senator Kay Bailey Hutchison of Texas as a "festering sore."[20]

In March 1996, at an international breast cancer conference in Falun, Sweden, updated results from the world's mammography screening trials were presented. Significantly, the Swedish Overview, a combined analysis of five separate Swedish trials, showed a 23 percent reduction in mortality for women under fifty, a result that was on the cusp of statistical significance. A combined analysis of all screening trials, excluding the Canadian Trial, showed a 24 percent mortality reduction, which *was* statistically significant.[21] NCI officials, including the new director, Richard Klausner, were in attendance and were impressed by the results. Klausner decided that it was time for the NCI to take a second bite of the controversial apple.

Shortly after Falun, plans were set in motion for a National Institutes of Health Consensus Development Conference. NIH Consensus Development Conferences are organized to resolve particularly difficult or controversial questions. They have been described as a sort of "science court" where experts on the topic under consideration make presentations to a panel brought together to "judge" the evidence. The aim typically is to assemble a diverse panel, reflecting all relevant interests, and construct a roster of speakers that is representative of the full spectrum of opinions on the subject. The more structured and formalized Consensus Development Conference approach was likely selected by Klausner because his predecessor, Samuel Broder, had been specifically criticized for using a more freewheeling workshop approach in the 1993 episode.[22] It is worth noting that the very first NIH Consensus Development Conference took place in 1977, and it was convened to resolve issues surrounding mammography in women under fifty in the BCDDP. Since then, there had been 102 such gatherings.

The NIH Consensus Development Conference on Breast Cancer Screening for Women Ages 40–49 was held January 21–23, 1997, at the NIH campus in Bethesda, Maryland. The panel initially consisted of thirteen members, including radiologists, oncologists, obstetrician/gynecologists, surgeons, statisticians, epidemiologists, and members of the advocacy community, one of whom was a breast cancer survivor.[23] There were seven women and six men. The panel chair was epidemiologist Leon Gordis of Johns Hopkins University School of Medicine. There was a palpable sense of high drama and expectancy among the over one thousand people who packed the auditorium where the conference was held. Backers of under-fifty screening wondered if the NIH and NCI would "get it right" this time.

The panel was charged with answering five key questions:

- Does screening reduce breast cancer mortality among women forty to forty-nine?
- What are the risks of screening?
- Are there any other benefits associated with screening?
- What is known about how the benefits and risks of screening differ according to a patient's risk factors?
- What are the directions for future research?

Over the course of a day and a half of testimony, the panel and audience heard presentations from thirty-two experts. Updated results from all eight randomized controlled trials were presented. Swedish researchers presented statistically significant mortality reductions among women forty to forty-nine in two of their five regional screening trials. Because the results in these two trials had achieved statistical significance, the Swedish Overview, which combined the results from all five trials, now showed a statistically significant 26 percent reduction in mortality. Finally, a new analysis combining the results of all randomized controlled trials, except the Canadian Trial, showed a statistically significant 23 percent reduction in mortality for women under fifty. In fact, because the new Swedish results were so strong, even when the Canadian findings were included, the results remained statistically significant at 16 percent.[24]

Given all the favorable new data that had been presented, it came as quite a surprise when the conference panel presented its draft statement on the final afternoon. The panel stated that current data "do not warrant a universal recommendation for mammography for all women in their forties. Each woman should decide for herself whether to undergo mammography."[25] Reaction was swift and forceful. One radiologist called the report "fraudulent."[26] Another characterized it as a "death sentence" for American women in their forties.[27] Even NCI director Klausner seemed flummoxed, expressing "shock" at the report.[28] Former NIH director Bernadine Healy would later deride the conference panel as "the Panel of Babel."[29]

In 1993 the issue for the NCI had been the lack of statistically significant mortality reductions for women under fifty in mammography screening trials. This time, with that standard having been met, other factors seemed to hold sway. Since the benefits to women aged forty to forty-nine did not appear, in any trial, until at least ten years after starting screening, the panel expressed concern that the benefit might actually be due to screening that occurred after study participants turned fifty, a phenomenon termed "age creep." Furthermore, panel members gave significant weight to the "risks" of screening, such as false positive and false negative readings, the possibility of radiation-induced breast cancer, and the overdiagnosis of low-risk, slow-growing cancers that might never have caused the patient any problems in her lifetime.

Even though, when the committee's draft report was unveiled, it was presented as a unanimous verdict, within days one panel member resigned in protest, citing concerns about the thrust of the report as it made its way through the revision process.[30] Two other members chose not to attach their names to the final report but issued a minority report instead. In it they criticized the majority for overemphasizing the "risks" of screening and minimizing the benefits. In the previous 102 Consensus Development Conferences hosted by the NIH since 1977, unanimous consent had been achieved in all but two instances.[31] As soon as the conference had completed its work, Klausner announced that the matter would be referred to the NCI's advisory panel, the National Cancer Advisory Board, at its next meeting in February 1997.

On February 4, 1997, in the U.S. Senate, a nonbinding resolution was proposed by Senator Olympia Snowe, Republican of Maine, and fifty-two co-sponsors, including all of the other female senators. It called on the National Cancer Advisory Board to consider reissuing the pre-1993 guideline for women forty to forty-nine and directed the public to adhere to screening guidelines issued by organizations other than the (U.S. government's own) NCI. The resolution was approved 98–0.[32]

The following day, Senator Arlen Spector, Republican of Pennsylvania and chairman of the powerful Subcommittee on Departments of Labor, Health and Human Services, and Education, and Related Agencies, which controls NIH funding, began a series of public hearings on the matter which continued into early March. In his opening remarks Specter made it clear that, although he was willing to listen to all sides of the issue, his mind was made up. "Ordinarily," he began, "we have these hearings to find the facts and decide what to do. I would say at the outset of this hearing that I have a fixed opinion on the subject, that women in their forties ought to be tested with mammograms."[33] His position seems to have stemmed from personal experience with a medical system that was more focused on containing costs than on doing what was best for the patient. He related a recent incident when he had had to demand an MRI scan from his unwilling doctors, only for it to show that he had a brain tumor. Others have surmised that his forcefulness on this issue was a continuing attempt to rehabilitate his image with female constituents after his harsh treatment of Anita Hill during the Clarence Thomas Supreme Court confirmation hearings six years earlier.[34] By the conclusion of the series of hearings, Specter expressed confidence "that we will be successful in having mammograms available to women 40–49."[35]

In March 1997 the American Cancer Society and the American College of Radiology updated their guidelines to recommend more aggressive screening for women in their forties. Both groups had previously recommended screening every one to two years. They now recommended annual screening for all women, beginning at age forty. The change was due to evidence that breast cancer grows more rapidly in premenopausal than in postmenopausal women. For screening to be effective, they reasoned, it needed to occur more frequently than every two years. In a thinly veiled swipe at the "Panel of Babel," the ACS proclaimed, "We make this recommendation forcefully, unambiguously and with no reservations," as it announced its new guidelines.[36]

Since the keeper of the NIH's purse strings had already declared confidence that the matter would soon be resolved to his liking, it should be no surprise that, barely a month later, the National Cancer Advisory Board had fully considered the issue and completed the process by mailed balloting. The final vote was 17–1 in favor of reissuing the pre-1993 guideline on screening women in their forties. These women would be advised to undergo screening every one to two years. NCI director Klausner announced that the NCI would immediately adopt the advisory board's recommendation. President Clinton also praised the new developments and pledged to work to ensure that federal health plans would cover screening mammography *annually*, beginning at age forty.[37]

(6)

PULLING THE PLUG ON GRANNY

The 1997 NIH-NCI episode had two far-reaching consequences. First, it established the primacy of politics over science in mammography disputes. No longer would science have the last word. If the conclusion based on scientific data was politically untenable, it would simply be overruled or circumvented by political leaders. This priority, evolving for about a decade, came to full fruition during this episode. Second, for the first time, a de facto U.S. government position on the screening of women under fifty was defined. Since that time the federal government has, despite the conclusions of its own scientific agencies, consistently been on the "pro" side in the under-fifty screening controversy. When, in the fall of 2009, mammography became embroiled yet again in controversy, these recently minted notions led to a swift resolution of the conflict. In fact, I will show why this may be the *last* time we have a heated national debate on mammography screening.

Mea Culpa

A very curious thing happened in October 2009. In a moment of unprecedented candor for an official of the normally message-disciplined American Cancer Society, Dr. Otis Brawley, its chief medical officer, made a startling admission in a *New York Times* interview: "We don't want people to panic but I'm admitting that American medicine has overpromised when it comes to screening. The advantages to screening have been exaggerated." He went on to say that even though mammography can save lives, "if a woman says, 'I don't want it,' I would not think badly of her but I'd like her to get it."[1]

Brawley was responding to an article recently published in the *Journal of the American Medical Association*.[2] In it, researchers made the argument that twenty years of widespread breast and prostate cancer screening had failed to deliver the promised health benefits. In the case of both diseases, population-based screening had resulted in a huge increase in the incidence of early stage disease with only a very slight decrease in late stage disease. This is significant because the basic rationale for screening has always been that identifying and treating more early stage cancers will result in a *commensurate* decrease in the number of late stage cancers and an overall improvement in the health status of the population. In other words, for every one hundred early stage breast cancers diagnosed, there should be one hundred fewer late stage cancers. This, however, has not been the case, suggesting that screening detects many non-aggressive cancers that would not have progressed if undetected and would have had no impact on the individual's life. The practical result of this has been a dramatic increase in the number of individuals treated for cancer without necessarily improving the health of the population, phenomena known as *overdiagnosis* and *overtreatment*. This 2009 article, widely reported on in the lay press, drew renewed attention to one of the potential downsides (harms) of screening and forced the ACS to acknowledge that its "one simple message (just do it!)" approach to mammography promotion may have done American women a disservice.

The Start of Rationing

The United States Preventive Services Task Force (USPSTF) is a federal agency that was established by the U.S. Public Health Service in 1984. It consists of panels of disinterested experts, charged with periodically reviewing the scientific justification underlying a wide array of clinical preventive services, including cancer screening. These services or activities are given letter grades (from A to D) meant to indicate the strength of the scientific evidence for a benefit associated with that particular activity. At this writing the USPSTF has a portfolio of over one hundred preventive activities for which it makes recommendations. These recommendations are updated every five years. Though not official government policy, USPSTF recommendations often inform public and private health policymaking.

On November 16, 2009, in a move that shocked government officials, medical professionals, and the lay public, the USPSTF published new, and very controversial, breast cancer screening guidelines.[3] These new guidelines, among other things, rescinded the group's recommendation for screening mammography for women younger than fifty, which had been in effect only since 2002. According to the USPSTF's analysis, screening mammography in women under fifty resulted in a 15 percent reduction in breast cancer mortality. While the Task Force found that this was the same mortality reduction enjoyed by women aged fifty to fifty-nine, it was significantly less than the 32 percent benefit seen in women sixty to sixty-nine. Furthermore, because breast cancer is less common in women under fifty, the group found that in order to avert one death from breast cancer, 1,904 women under fifty, as opposed to 1,339 women fifty to fifty-nine and 377 women sixty to sixty-nine, would have to be screened. The Task Force also gave significant consideration to the possible *harms* of screening mammography. The panel members considered radiation exposure, pain, anxiety, false positive or false negative results, and overdiagnosis potentially important harms. Their analysis showed that women under fifty were much more likely than other age groups to receive a false positive mammogram. This is an abnormal report that requires additional mammography or ultrasound for a finding that is ultimately determined to be trivial. With this in mind, the Task Force adopted the following position: "The USPSTF recommends against routine screening mammography in women aged 40–49 years. The decision to start regular, biennial screening mammography before the age of 50 years should be an individual one and take into account patient context, including the patient's values regarding specific benefits and harms. (Grade C recommendation)."[4]

Though the panel's recommendation had been voted on in the summer of 2008, its official publication date was dictated by the publishing schedule of the medical journal in which it was to be released. The timing could not have been worse. The political climate in the United States in the latter half of 2009 was particularly raw and toxic. Congress was in the midst of debating the Affordable Care Act, the Obama administration's effort at reforming the U.S. health care system. That summer, in town hall meetings all across the country, members of Congress had faced loud and hostile constituents opposed to this legislation. The national conversation about the proposed law devolved into ominous warnings about "death panels" and "pulling the plug on granny." Thus, it should be no surprise that the new USPSTF mammography guidelines were immediately denounced as the first example of the coming of health care rationing. "This is how rationing begins. This is the little toe in the edge of the water. This is when you start getting a bureaucrat between you and your physician," Representative Marsha Blackburn, a Tennessee Republican, was quoted as saying.[5] Congressional Republicans and other critics of the health care reform legislation frequently pointed to language in the Senate version of the bill that required health plans to cover only those preventive services that received an A or B rating from the USPSTF.

Mammography's most reliable defenders quickly mounted a full-throated condemnation of the Task Force. The American College of Radiology issued a press release in which it characterized the USPSTF guidelines as "a step backward and . . . a significant harm to women's health." The chair of the organization's board of chancellors, Dr. James A. Thrall, saw these developments as a "move toward a new health care rationing policy that will turn back the clock on medicine for decades."[6] He called on the secretary of Health and Human Services, Kathleen Sebelius, to *order* the USPSTF to rescind its guidelines.[7] The ACS's Brawley, despite his public mea culpa just one month earlier, bemoaned the ongoing criticism of mammography. "How many mothers, sisters, aunts, grandmothers, daughters and friends are we willing to lose to breast cancer while the debate goes on about the limitations of mammography?" he wrote in a *Washington Post* op-ed piece.[8]

Not only was the USPSTF's report widely panned, but also its sixteen-member panel endured repeated ad hominem attacks. By design, USPSTF panels are constituted in such a way as to limit potential conflicts of interest. For that reason there were no radiologists on the panel, although radiologists outside the panel participated in the peer review of the panel's work. This absence of radiologists (imaging experts) on the panel was used to disparage the qualifications and expertise of the panel as a whole. In a CNN interview, Harvard Medical School radiologist Daniel Kopans was dismissive of the USPSTF panelists: "I know all the experts in the United States in mammography screening and all the ones around the world. I don't know any of these people."[9] It didn't particularly help their case, however, that panel members who did television interviews did not always come across as confident or authoritative. It was clear that they had been caught completely off guard by the controversy that had engulfed their work. Panel vice chair Dr. Diane Petitti admitted in a *New York Times* interview that she was unacquainted with the long history of controversy surrounding the appropriateness of mammography in women under fifty. "I was relatively unaware of it. I have been made aware of it now," she is reported to have said.[10] In its twenty-five-year existence the USPSTF had issued hundreds of guidelines on scores of subjects. Most had received no media attention whatsoever. None had ever received this type of public denunciation.

The advocacy community was divided on this issue. Nancy G. Brinker, founder of Susan G. Komen for the Cure, predicted "mass confusion and justifiable outrage" over the new screening recommendations.[11] Fran Visco, president of the National Breast Cancer Coalition, welcomed the new guidelines, arguing that there had been too much emphasis on avoiding confusion and providing women with an unambiguous message on screening. "We would argue that that, while messages need to be simple, they need to be truthful. Women deserve the facts," she said.[12] Dr. Susan Love, the renowned breast surgeon and founder and president of the Susan Love Research Foundation, strongly supported the USPSTF, both on her blog and in a round of media interviews. For example, on *Good Morning America*, Love stated categorically that mammography had "never been shown to work in women under fifty" and furthermore confessed, "We've sort of oversold the notion of early detection."[13] Love's vocal support for the new screening regimen led to a deluge of angry messages posted on her blog site, including one that screamed bluntly, "Have you lost your freakin' mind?"[14] This was apparently so distressing that in her next blog post she found it necessary to declare, "I had nothing to do with formulating these guidelines" and "I have not been influenced [by] or received any donations from any insurance companies, nor have I been bought off by our federal government."[15]

These few voices of support notwithstanding, public opinion was overwhelmingly against the USPSTF's new recommendations. A USA Today–Gallup poll, conducted in the days following the release of the new mammography guidelines, found that 76 percent of women aged thirty-five to seventy-five disagreed with the USPSTF, including 47 percent who *strongly* disagreed.[16] Eighty-four percent of women aged thirty-five to forty-nine planned to ignore the recommendations altogether and continue having mammograms before fifty. Most significantly, 76 percent of respondents believed that the new screening protocol had been proposed for its cost savings. Only 16 percent believed that the decision was based on an assessment of the risks and benefits of the procedure. Thus, even though it had been widely reported that the USPSTF's review of its mammography guidelines had begun in 2007 under the George W. Bush administration, and that the vote to adopt the new screening schedule was taken in July 2008, months before the presidential election, in the public's mind the illusory dots between "Obamacare," health care rationing, and the USPSTF mammography guidelines had now been completely connected.

The Obama administration, which had come to power stressing a new respect for science and the depoliticization of the scientific process, found itself in a quandary: accept the advice of this government-appointed panel of independent scientific experts and watch its health care reform effort go down in defeat, or reject it and risk comparisons to the Bush administration in its handling of the controversy surrounding government-sponsored stem cell research. The decision came quickly. Within forty-eight hours of the USPSTF's announcement, Health and Human Services secretary Kathleen Sebelius publicly disavowed its recommendations. In a November 18, 2009, statement, Sebelius commented:

The US Preventive (Services) Task Force is an outside, independent panel of doctors and scientists who make recommendations. They do not set federal policy and they don't determine what services are covered by the federal government. . . . [O]ur policies remain unchanged. Indeed I would be very surprised if any private insurance company changed its mammography coverage decisions as a result of this action. . . . My message is simple. Mammograms have always been an important life-saving tool in the fight against breast cancer and they still are today. Keep doing what you have been doing for years.[17]

Democrats in Congress were in a slightly more comfortable position than the White House. Their tradition of strong support for women's health issues dovetailed nicely with their desire to get the Affordable Care Act passed. They had made no promise to be deferential to science. In December 2009 the House of Representatives unanimously passed a nonbinding resolution, sponsored by Representative Debbie Wasserman Schultz, a Florida Democrat and herself a breast cancer survivor, admonishing private insurers not to attempt to use the new USPSTF guidelines to deny mammography coverage for women under fifty.[18] That same month, the Health Subcommittee of the House Energy and Commerce Committee, chaired by Representative Frank Pallone, a Democrat from New Jersey, held a day-long hearing into the circumstances surrounding the USPSTF affair.[19]

In the Senate, an amendment to the evolving new health care law, sponsored by Senator Barbara Mikulski, a Maryland Democrat, won easy approval. Its language was direct: "The Secretary [of Health and Human Services] shall not use any recommendation made by the United States Preventive Services Task Force to deny coverage of an item or service by a group health plan or health insurance issuer offering group or individual health insurance coverage or under a Federal health care program or private insurance."[20]

All That Is Old Is New Again

In the end, the controversy died a quick death. Political leaders moved on to the final push to pass the Affordable Care Act.

Once that was done, the Department of Health and Human Services made it official: the 2009 USPSTF guidelines would simply be ignored. In a July 2010 press release the department formally announced that under the Affordable Care Act, insurers would be required to cover screening mammography in accordance with the USPSTF's old (2002) guidelines, which recommended routine screening beginning at age forty (grade B by USPSTF rankings). Essentially, the *old* guidelines were now *current* and the new guidelines were given an early retirement. Furthermore, the department would convene a *new* panel of (non-USPSTF) experts to bring forth revised (and presumably more politically acceptable) guidelines.[21] In October 2010, in his annual Breast Cancer Awareness Month proclamation, President Obama reiterated this message: "For women ages 40 and over, regular mammograms and clinical breast exams . . . every one to two years are the most effective way to find breast cancer early, when it may be easier to treat. . . . The Affordable Care Act, which I was proud to sign into law earlier this year, requires all new health insurance policies to cover recommended preventive service, without any additional cost, including annual mammogram screenings for women over 40."[22]

The End of the Fight?

It is highly probable that we have witnessed the *final* major national debate on screening mammography. I make this argument for the following reasons. First, the underlying science is not likely to change. Mammography has been studied in excruciating detail. After many large scientific trials and real-life experience spanning the past forty years and more, we know what the answers are. Screening mammography reduces deaths from breast cancer. This is true for all women over forty, but the effect is greater for women over fifty (postmenopausal). Screening mammography has certain risks, and some of these are more common in women under fifty.

Furthermore, since the likelihood of breast cancer increases with age, the risk-benefit calculus becomes more favorable as women age. These basic facts are unlikely to change in the future. Second, the fight over screening women under fifty has always been about *access*. Lack of insurance coverage for screening mammography is a known barrier that keeps women from being tested. It is clear that, at both the federal and state levels, political leaders have made the decision that American women have a right to screening mammography starting at age forty. Given the fact that the science is now mature and unlikely to change, one is hard-pressed to envision a scenario in which political leaders would ever consider rolling back insurance coverage mandates. Without a threat to access, another major fracas is unlikely to arise. The position of screening mammography is secure until a replacement technology comes along.

(7)

THE HOUSE
THAT MAMMOGRAPHY BUILT

With a little help from its friends, screening mammography has not merely survived its myriad controversies, it has thrived. Eighty-one percent of women over fifty and 65 percent of women forty to forty-nine undergo regular screening.[1] As mammography succeeded, a vast multifaceted collateral economy developed around it. In this screening-centric system, the various elements in the secondary economy are directly sustained by ongoing screening. This remarkable phenomenon, without ready parallel, is the subject of this chapter.

When Mammography Fails:
The Demand for Legal Recourse

Over the past few decades of widespread screening mammography, countless lives have been saved. But there is also a large population of women for whom mammography failed. "Saves" and "misses": these are the everyday realities of life with an imperfect test. As noted in an insurance industry report on breast cancer litigation, as screening rates increase, "there are increased opportunities for both diagnosis and misdiagnosis of breast cancer."[2]

Screening mammography has largely been promoted with simple, direct messages. In fact, simplicity of message, in order to avoid public confusion, has been the overriding consideration in most mammography public awareness campaigns. These simple messages have been justifiably criticized on two points. First, they have often utilized images of young (premenopausal) women, thereby needlessly heightening fear of the disease in women of this demographic while masking the reality that breast cancer is much more common later in life.[3] Second, they have tended to overemphasize the potential benefits of screening while remaining largely silent on its limitations. The statement "Mammography can find breast cancer as small as the period at the end of this sentence" appeared on many promotional materials in the 1980s and 1990s. As a result, many women significantly overestimate the capabilities of mammography.[4] In a 2003 international survey, 45 percent of American women stated a belief that more than one hundred breast cancer deaths would be prevented if one thousand women underwent screening for ten years. Only 3 percent of respondents were able to identify the correct answer, stated by the study's authors to be five deaths per every thousand women screened.[5] Not only do American women overestimate the mortality-reducing benefits of mammography, but also a majority harbor the belief that mammography actually *prevents* breast cancer from occurring. In fact, for many women the term "screening" is synonymous with "prevention." Some screening tests can in fact prevent or reduce the likelihood of getting the disease being screened for. For example, removing polyps during screening colonoscopy prevents many cases of colon cancer. Mammography, however, reduces the risk of *dying* of breast cancer by finding it earlier. It does not prevent or reduce the chances of *getting* the disease the way that colonoscopy does for colon cancer. The public has never been educated on this nuance. As a result, according to that same 2003 survey, 57 percent of American women believed that mammography prevents or reduces the risk of *contracting* breast cancer.[6] Thus it is not surprising that when breast cancer occurs in a woman who has religiously adhered to a regimen of annual mammography, both she and her loved ones are shocked, angry, and confused. This is especially true for cases in which the mammogram was misinterpreted.

In the mid-1990s, when routine screening mammography was becoming widely practiced, delay in diagnosing breast cancer became the most common reason for patients to file medical malpractice lawsuits. It has maintained this status ever since. During the period 1995–2001, claims totaled over $170 million. In these cases radiologists were the most frequently named defendants and mammogram misinterpretation the most common allegation. Even though breast cancer is much more common in postmenopausal women, the vast majority (68 percent) of claimants were women under the age of fifty.[7] Thus, ironically, radiologists, who have been among the most vocal backers of expanded screening of younger women, are the principal recipients of those patients' ire when mammography fails.

Testing Begets Testing: The Demand for More

Although mammography *is* effective in reducing the death rate from breast cancer, it is far from a perfect test. It raises many red flags over findings that are not cancer (false positives); it misses up to 15 percent of cancers that are present (false negatives); and, as mentioned in the previous chapter, some of the cancers it does find would have had no impact on the woman's life if left undetected (overdiagnosis). These limitations have, among other things, driven demand for a variety of other imaging tests and procedures. In this regard, mammography has been characterized by the sociologist and women's health researcher Patricia Kaufert as an economic "demand generator."[8]

False Positives

On a mammogram, it is not always clear what is cancer and what is not. There is a great deal of overlap in the appearance of cancer and noncancerous abnormalities. A smooth, round lump in one woman may represent a benign tumor; an identical-looking smooth round lump in another woman may be breast cancer. This lack of specificity results in a large number of screened women being recalled for additional evaluation. The *screening recall rate* is the percentage of women who are given an abnormal reading and asked to undergo additional testing. In the United States this rate is 10 to 15 percent. In Europe, where radiologists do not live with the pervasive threat of medical malpractice litigation that U.S. radiologists face, it is about half that figure.[9] The vast majority (95 percent) of screening-detected abnormalities are ultimately found to be noncancerous (false positives). On average, for every 1,000 American women who undergo screening, 100 to 150 are recalled for additional imaging. Of these, about twenty to twenty-five will be advised to have a biopsy, and about five cancers will be found. After ten years of screening, starting at age forty, an American woman has a 61 percent chance of a false positive result.[10]

The additional testing after an abnormal mammogram typically involves specialized mammography views or ultrasound but may also include a biopsy. As routine screening gained widespread acceptance in the late 1980s to 1990s, there was a huge increase in the number of small (non-palpable) breast abnormalities requiring biopsy. This led to the development of non-surgical breast biopsy approaches, such as stereotactic and ultrasound-guided core needle biopsy, which could be performed in the mammography center. These techniques use a modified mammogram machine or ultrasound, respectively, to help guide a needle into the abnormal tissue for biopsy. They have all but replaced surgical biopsy as the first diagnostic step following the identification of a suspicious breast abnormality.

For every $100 spent on screening, an additional $30 to $33 is spent to evaluate false positive findings.[11] In the Medicare population, it is estimated that the workup of false positive mammogram results is a $250 million annual expense.[12]

There is a strong consensus on the value of cancer screening among the American public. In a 2004 national survey of 500 men and women, 87 percent agreed with the statement "cancer screening tests for healthy persons are almost always a good idea."[13] This widespread belief in the benefits of screening comes from our collective acceptance of the early detection message that has been widely promoted over the past several decades, direct-to-consumer marketing of screening tests by commercial enterprises, and our persistent primal fear of cancer. In that same 2004 survey, 66 percent of respondents stated their desire to be screened even for cancers for which there is no treatment and 65 percent felt that there would never be a time in their life when it would be appropriate to discontinue screening.[14] For many, cancer screening is a "moral obligation." About 75 percent of survey participants felt that a fifty-five-year-old woman who did not undergo screening mammography was "irresponsible." An eighty-year-old woman not having mammograms was deemed "irresponsible" by 41 percent.[15]

Because the belief in screening is so profound, acceptance of false positives, as an unavoidable by-product, is high. Although over 90 percent of women who have had a false-positive mammogram rate the experience as "scary," 96 percent report being happy that they had the test, and 90 percent continue to have mammograms as often as or more frequently than before.[16] When asked how many false positive mammogram results are acceptable for each life saved, 63 percent of women would tolerate 500 or more and 37 percent would tolerate 10,000 or more.[17]

False Negatives

Mammography misses up to 15 percent of breast cancers. Its effectiveness is particularly limited in women with dense breasts. On a mammogram, breast tissue may appear to be composed primarily of white tissue (dense breasts), dark gray tissue (fatty breasts), or some combination of the two. Typically, premenopausal women have dense breasts and older women have more fatty breasts. Dense breast tissue is particularly problematic because on a mammogram, breast cancer appears as a white object. Thus the whiter the tissue, the more difficult it is to identify a white object within it. Finding a polar bear in a snowstorm is a commonly used analogy. Much of the mammography-driven new technology has been developed to address this issue. For example, computer-aided detection (CAD) uses a computer program to assist the radiologist in identifying breast cancer. Though CAD may improve radiologist performance, it also raises many erroneous red flags and results in higher rates of screening recall and biopsy.[18]

Because the vast majority of lumps found on mammography do not represent cancer, ultrasound has become an indispensible tool in breast imaging. Many women have an ultrasound after an abnormal mammogram to distinguish between a trivial fluid-filled cyst and a potentially serious solid mass. Ultrasound has an additional strength in that, unlike mammography, it is not degraded by dense breast tissue. A few studies have examined whether ultrasound should be used as an additional *screening* test in women who have dense breasts. They have shown that more cancers are found by screening with both tests as opposed to mammography alone. Ultrasound, however, finds a great many noncancerous lumps, so women who undergo this "double screening" regimen have many more unnecessary (false positive) biopsies than their mammography-alone counterparts.[19]

Similarly, breast MRI (magnetic resonance imaging) has achieved a prominent place in breast imaging. It finds many more breast cancers than does mammography but also suffers from high rates of false positives. Furthermore, relative to mammography and ultrasound, it is extremely expensive and, until recently, has not been widely available. For these reasons it is not considered a good screening test for women at average risk. In 2007 the American Cancer Society recommended that women at *extremely* high risk of breast cancer (for example, those who have the BRCA1 or BRCA2 genetic mutations) undergo annual screening with MRI in addition to mammography.[20]

The story of Nancy Cappello is an apt illustration of the theme of this section. In 2004 the Woodbury, Connecticut, resident came face-to-face with one of mammography's major flaws. Cappello, a fifty-two-year-old education consultant with no family history of breast cancer, was diagnosed with advanced breast cancer two months after a "normal" mammogram report. Her tumor was noted in a routine physical and subsequently confirmed on an ultrasound. She was shocked to find out later that she had dense breast tissue and that not only had this made her mammogram more prone to missing breast cancer but also her risk of developing breast cancer was actually greater than for women with fatty breast tissue. Calling this mammography's "best kept secret," she later founded an organization, Are You Dense? dedicated to educating women about dense breast tissue and advocating for legislation promoting screening with ultrasound.[21]

In 2006 Connecticut, under Governor Jodi M. Rell, herself a breast cancer survivor, became the first state to mandate insurance coverage for *screening* breast ultrasound (in addition to mammography) for women with dense breast tissue.[22] Recognizing that most women with dense breast tissue are not aware of it, Cappello and her allies pushed state political leaders to pass patient notification legislation. In 2009, in another national first, Connecticut enacted legislation requiring mammography facilities to inform patients about their breast density. The law mandated that patient notification letters include the following language: "If your mammogram demonstrates that you have dense breast tissue, which could hide small abnormalities, you might benefit from supplementary screening tests, which can include a breast ultrasound screening or a breast MRI examination, or both."[23] The new law aimed to increase utilization of the supplemental tests by making sure that women in the target demographic were so informed. Similar legislation was soon pending in several other states. In 2011, Texas became the second state in the nation to enact breast-density patient-notification legislation.[24] Later that year, a similar law, passed by the California legislature, was vetoed by Gov. Jerry Brown.[25] Density Education National Survivors' Effort (DENSE), an organization Cappello co-founded, is pushing to nationalize the Connecticut model through federal legislation.[26] Currently, approximately 37 million screening mammograms are performed in the United States every year.[27] Overall, no more than 10 percent of mammograms reveal breasts that are completely fatty. Thus, at least 90 percent of mammograms show some amount of dense tissue that could potentially mask breast cancer.[28] Should the Connecticut law be replicated at the federal level, breast cancer screening would potentially be transformed from 37 million mammograms to 37 million mammograms *plus* 33 million (37 million x 90 percent) ultrasounds annually. Given Medicare reimbursement rates ($131 for mammography, $89 for ultrasound), this would increase annual expenditures from $4.8 billion to $7.7 billion. This figure does not even include the costs associated with the additional unnecessary biopsies generated by the (unavoidable) false positive ultrasound scans.

The Little *Pink* Engine: The Demand for Everything

There are 2.5 million breast cancer survivors in the United States today. This is a larger cohort than for any other cancer. Of these

2.5 million women, 500,000 carry a diagnosis of stage 0 breast cancer, otherwise known as ductal carcinoma in situ. As I noted earlier, DCIS is a disease that was practically unheard of prior to the advent of screening mammography. Now it constitutes 20 to 25 percent of all new breast cancer diagnoses. This condition is poorly understood. It is widely believed that as many as one third to one half of all such abnormalities would never progress to lethal *invasive* breast cancer if left alone.[29] Yet because of our inability to distinguish the good actors from the potentially bad actors, all patients diagnosed with DCIS receive treatment for breast cancer. DCIS was partly responsible for the "epidemic" narrative that developed around breast cancer in the late 1980s to early 1990s, just as screening mammography was becoming widely practiced. In fact, former first lady Nancy Reagan was diagnosed with a tiny, mammographically detected DCIS breast cancer in 1987.

It was in the midst of the mammography-driven breast cancer "epidemic" that breast cancer cause-related marketing was born. "Cause-related marketing" is a phrase that was coined and trademarked by American Express in 1983. In that year the company embarked on an innovative marketing strategy aimed at increasing credit card usage. It partnered with the Statue of Liberty–Ellis Island Foundation, Inc., in a three-month campaign. During that period, whenever a card member made a purchase with the American Express credit card, the company donated one dollar toward the Statue of Liberty restoration effort. Not only was American Express able to donate $1.7 million to the cause, but also card usage increased by 27 percent and new applications jumped by 45 percent. This was the first demonstration that corporate alignment with an esteemed social cause could be an effective means of boosting sales.[30] Cause-related marketing is not the same as corporate philanthropy in which a company donates money to a nonprofit organization without expecting anything return. Rather it is, at its heart, a marketing strategy whereby the company enhances its public image (the halo effect) and drives consumers to its products by affiliating itself with a favored cause or issue.[31]

Nancy G. Brinker, founder of the Susan G. Komen Breast Cancer Foundation (now Susan G. Komen for the Cure), is widely regarded as the prime mover in the evolution of breast cancer cause-related marketing. The foundation, launched in 1982, was named for Brinker's sister, who, two years earlier, had lost a painful battle to breast cancer at the age of thirty-six. The organization is best known for its annual charity 5K event, Race for the Cure. Started in Dallas in 1983, Race for the Cure events take place in over one hundred U.S. cities and several foreign countries, attracting 1.5 million participants annually. Brinker's early forays into the world of cause-related marketing were largely rebuffed. In 1984 she made several unsuccessful bids to persuade New York lingerie manufacturers to allow Komen to place breast cancer informational hang tags on their bras. One executive, upon hearing Brinker's sales pitch, is reported to have emphatically declared: "No. No, no. We want women to feel happy and sexy when they think of our product. We're selling beauty and femininity. You're selling disease and death."[32]

By 1989, however, as fear of the new breast cancer "epidemic" was on the rise, Susan G. Komen successfully signed its first corporate sponsorship deal. New Balance Athletic Shoe, Inc., became a national sponsor of Race for the Cure. In addition to being a race sponsor, the company has operated an in-store promotion, Lace Up for the Cure, in which 5 percent of the proceeds from the sale of select footwear is donated to Komen. At this writing Komen has 240 corporate partners, including the eleven members of its Million Dollar Council Elite, each of which pledges to donate $1 million annually. These corporate relationships add over $50 million to Komen's annual fund-raising tally.[33]

Susan G. Komen for the Cure, though not without its critics, is a generally well regarded charity that has earned the highest four-star rating from Charity Navigator. In its twenty-five years of existence, it has donated $1.5 billion to breast cancer research and to early detection and awareness efforts.[34] Beyond the work of Komen and other respected, transparent advocacy organizations, every October an immense, nebulous pink tide rolls in over American retail for Breast Cancer Awareness Month. Suddenly, products from makeup to vacuum cleaners, breath mints to jewelry, and fast food to kitchen appliances appear sporting the little pink ribbon and vague promises to support breast cancer awareness or other efforts. My personal favorite is the trademarked Pink Ribbon Bagel available at my local bakery. This is a delightful little cherry-filled, ribbon-shaped, soft, chewy bagel with a pinkish hue that is oh so good! It costs more than the other bagels on the rack (naturally), but I happily hand over the extra cash to enjoy the rare treat. Never once have I bothered to ask how much, if any, of the extra cost is donated to breast cancer–related causes. Though I consider myself relatively well informed on this issue, my sweet tooth makes me a cause marketer's dream consumer. Assume you're helping the cause, pay the higher price, and ask no questions.

Breast cancer cause-related marketing has benefited from mammography screening in three principal ways. First, it was the mammography-induced breast cancer "epidemic" of 1987–1991 that led to the emergence of a new wave of activism which drew the attention of the nation and its political leaders to this disease. One wonders whether the numerous major accomplishments of this period would have been possible without the focusing effect of this statistical epiphenomenon. It certainly provided an appropriate milieu for the concept of cause marketing to a population anxious about breast cancer to take hold.

As noted earlier, one fifth of the 2.5 million breast cancer survivors in the United States carry a diagnosis of ductal carcinoma in situ. In fact, over fifty thousand women receive this diagnosis each year. If, as is suspected, a large proportion of these cases would never have become harmful to the patient, then there are, potentially, tens of thousands of American women who fall into the category of screening-induced overdiagnosis every year. For every woman diagnosed with breast cancer, there are, at a conservative estimate, an additional twenty people—family, close friends, co-workers, and others—who are "touched" by the diagnosis. Thus, mammography's overdiagnosis problem tends to enlarge the population of "survivors and those who love them." These are the individuals who are most likely to be influenced by pink marketing.

Finally, the frequent, well-publicized mammography controversies over the past twenty years and more have kept breast cancer a "hot topic" in the public square. In this way, the cause marketer's aim of keeping the consumer thinking about the product and its association with the cause is greatly furthered.

(8)

OVERDIAGNOSIS: MAMMOGRAPHY'S BURDEN

In this final chapter I expand on a subject that was previously mentioned in passing. Mammography-induced breast cancer overdiagnosis represents the most significant detriment of screening. Yet until recently it has received almost no mention in the public education messages of government, advocacy, or professional entities. This deafening silence reflects the long-standing aversion of the pro-screening community to any public discussion of mammography's limitations. We have been afraid of "confusing" women with "mixed messages" on screening. This fear has prevented us from having the frank, honest conversations that are absolutely essential for genuine patient-consumer education to occur.

Seeking and Finding

As noted by health care sociologist Maren Klawiter, the mid-1980s transformation of mammography from a diagnostic test for women with breast symptoms to a screening test for *all* women represented a shift of the "mammographic gaze" into the vast untapped population of healthy women. As this occurred, the "Do Not Delay" message of early detection, promoted through the first three quarters of the twentieth century, morphed into a "Go in Search" admonition.[1] This new dogma would come to rely on increasingly sophisticated technology to find breast cancer in its embryonic stages. Under the earlier dispensation, breast cancer was to be treated as soon as it came to light. In the new order, it was to be sought out in the shadows.

Overdiagnosis refers to the identification of indolent or low-potential cancers that, absent screening, would not have become evident during the individual's lifetime. As elegantly described by H. Gilbert Welch and William C. Black, overdiagnosis occurs when a cancer is diagnosed that either (1) does not progress, or possibly even regresses; or (2) progresses so slowly that the individual dies of some other cause before ever developing symptoms.[2] In either case, these are cancers that, frankly, didn't need to be found. They are sometimes referred to as *pseudo-disease.* The idea that there are some cancers that don't need to be sought out and eliminated is difficult for laypeople, and even some professionals, to grasp. It is, however, a phenomenon that has been repeatedly observed throughout the history of cancer screening. Lung cancer (through screening chest X-rays for smokers), prostate cancer (through the prostate-specific antigen, or PSA, blood test), and breast cancer have been shown to be particularly prone to overdiagnosis.[3] Largely because of this issue, the U.S. Preventive Services Task Force in late 2011 dropped its recommendation for PSA testing in men younger than seventy-five years old, giving this practice a "D" rating (PSA testing in men older than seventy-five years already was rated "D")[4]

That a book about the social and political history of mammography should contain an entire chapter on overdiagnosis may seem overly pessimistic or even disparaging. But I am not pessimistic about mammography, nor is it my intent to denigrate it. My aim is simply to promote a wider understanding, and perhaps spark a debate on this critical subject. Overdiagnosis and mammography are inextricably linked. Apart from the effect in reducing breast cancer mortality, overdiagnosis has been screening mammography's most consequential legacy. Screening-related overdiagnosis contributed to the breast cancer "epidemic" of the late 1980s to early 1990s. It was this phenomenon, and society's response to it, that made fighting breast cancer the most favored disease cause and mammography the most favored weapon in the fight.

The DCIS Bubble

As I mentioned earlier, ductal carcinoma in situ (DCIS, also called intraductal carcinoma or stage 0 breast cancer) represents a stage of the disease in which the cancer cells are completely confined to the interior of the milk ducts. In fact the term "in situ" literally means that the tumor cells are still in their "original" location. Because the cancer cells have not breached the duct walls, typically there is no lump or other noticeable symptom associated with this disease. As long as the tumor remains confined to the milk ducts, there is no potential for it to spread beyond the breast and essentially no lethality. DCIS has a ten-year survival rate of 98 percent. This is in contrast to *invasive* (or infiltrating) breast cancer, in which the tumor is no longer confined to the interior of the milk ducts but has spread to the surrounding tissue. At this stage in development, it may form a lump that can be felt or may demonstrate some other sign or symptom. Invasive breast cancer has the potential to spread beyond the breast and can have lethal consequences. Although there is evidence of mammography-driven overdiagnosis of *both* invasive cancer and DCIS, the DCIS problem is much more straightforward and is the focus of this discussion.

DCIS is a disease that was largely unknown prior to the era of mammographic screening. Prior to mammography, DCIS constituted about 1 to 2 percent of breast cancer diagnoses.[5] Those few pre-mammography DCIS patients typically sought medical attention because of a lump or nipple discharge. Mastectomy was the treatment, and it was essentially curative.

Even though DCIS was uncommonly diagnosed in the pre-mammography era, there has always been a large reservoir of occult, or hidden, DCIS lesions within the breasts of healthy, asymptomatic women. The results of autopsy studies done on women who died of a variety of non–breast cancer causes suggest that up to 39 percent of women in the mammography age range (forty to seventy) may have DCIS and are unaware of it.[6]

It turns out that mammography is almost tailor-made for identifying DCIS. Many of these small, unsuspected DCIS lesions contain crystals of calcium salts, which appear on mammography as clusters of white specks that are commonly referred to as microcalcifications. These are relatively easy to identify, even in women who have dense breast tissue. In fact, whereas mammography may miss up to 25 percent of invasive breast cancers, it misses only about 14 percent of DCIS.[7]

The widespread use of screening mammography has resulted in an explosion of DCIS cases. There was a greater than sevenfold increase in the incidence rate of DCIS between 1980 (five cases per 100,000 women) and 1998 (thirty-seven cases per 100,000 women).[8] Currently, DCIS accounts for 20 to 25 percent of all new breast cancer cases, with fifty to sixty thousand new cases diagnosed annually. It has been estimated that one in every 1,300 mammography examinations results in a diagnosis of DCIS.[9] Over 500,000 American women are living with this diagnosis today.

For all the DCIS that has been diagnosed over the past quarter century, very little is known about its behavior and natural tendencies. We have employed a strategy of aggressively seeking out and treating DCIS in the hope that by identifying and treating cancer in this early stage, we can lower the incidence of invasive cancer. In other words, there should be a decrease in the incidence of invasive breast cancer proportional to the dramatic rise in DCIS rates. This has not occurred. Early stage invasive breast cancer incidence rates have remained high, and late stage invasive breast cancer rates have dipped only slightly, during the decades of the DCIS bubble.[10]

The reason for this is simple. While it is true that most invasive breast cancers first pass through a DCIS phase, the reverse is *not* also true. Most DCIS cases *do not* progress to invasive breast cancer. In fact, it is believed that only one third to one half of DCIS cases, left untreated, would progress to invasive cancer.[11] DCIS that does not progress to invasive cancer is completely harmless, having no lethal potential. It is a disease the individual will die *with* rather than die *from*. In this regard, a significant portion of mammographically detected DCIS potentially represents overdiagnosis.

There is as yet no reliable method of separating the harmless DCIS cases (those that will not progress to invasive cancer) from the potentially more dangerous ones (those that will progress). Because of this uncertainty, essentially all women who receive this diagnosis undergo cancer therapy. *Overtreatment* is thus the main hazard of overdiagnosis. The overdiagnosed cannot benefit from treatment, since in reality their cancers would not have caused a problem in their lifetime. They are, however, subject to the potential risks of treatment. The majority of women diagnosed with DCIS undergo lumpectomy, either with or without radiation therapy. Just under one third undergo mastectomy.[12] There is also a very troubling trend toward bilateral (double) mastectomy. Between 1998 and 2005, the proportion of DCIS patients choosing to have both breasts removed for preventive reasons more than doubled, from 2.1 percent to 5.2 percent.[13]

To date there has been no definitive proof that detecting large numbers of DCIS cases in a population of healthy women is beneficial. The mortality-reducing benefit of screening mammography occurs primarily through identifying small *invasive* cancers rather than in removing DCIS from the population. As the distinguished radiologist Lazlo Tabar and colleagues conclude, "compared with downward stage-shifting of invasive tumors [that is, detecting *invasive* tumors at smaller and smaller sizes], detection of DCIS plays a small part in saving lives from breast cancer."[14] In a 2011 article, the Harvard Medical School radiologist Daniel Kopans, arguably mammography's most vociferous proponent, conceded, "Unfortunately, at this point in time it is not possible to determine the contribution, if any, of the detection and treatment of DCIS lesions."[15] Thus the practical effect of our DCIS-detecting efforts of the past several decades has been to create a huge new class of women who receive a breast cancer diagnosis, along with all of its social, financial, and emotional accompaniments. These women are started on a pathway that involves disfiguring surgery for all, a long course of high-dose radiation for many, and treatment complications for some.

There is no ready solution to mammography's DCIS problem. Screening for breast cancer using mammography will inevitably lead to large numbers of DCIS cases being identified. Furthermore, not all DCIS is trivial. What is needed, however, is a change in our knee-jerk approach to this condition, which encourages and even requires radiologists to find as much of it as possible and surgeons to treat all of it aggressively. As Laura Esserman and Ian Thompson urge: "What we need now is a coming together of physicians and scientists of all disciplines to reduce the burden of cancer death AND cancer diagnosis. . . . By changing our clinical and scientific priorities to focus on distinguishing indolent from aggressive disease, we can improve the value of screening, reduce morbidity of treatment, and prevent lethal outcomes of cancer."[16]

What we call this condition may need to change. There are many influential voices in the scientific community who suggest that the word "carcinoma" should be dropped from the name entirely. In an interview following a 2009 National Institutes of Health state-of-the-science conference on DCIS, Dr. Otis Brawley, an oncologist and chief medical officer of the American Cancer Society, argued in support of a name change: "I'm much more concerned that we are scaring a whole host of people that have ductal carcinoma in situ who make rash decisions because it's called 'carcinoma'—decisions that they wouldn't make if it was more adequately described for what it truly is."[17] One proposed moniker, "IDLE tumor" (InDolent Lesions of Epithelial Origin) highlights the sluggishness of many of these lesions.[18]

The way physicians talk to patients about DCIS also needs to change. When a physician informs a patient that her breast biopsy has revealed DCIS, it is common for the information to be framed in a "this is really good news" construct. In this communication the patient is likely to be told that mammography found her cancer in the earliest possible stage, and that she should be quite pleased about this. There is often little to no discussion of the biological uncertainty of this condition and the lack of clarity about the best way to treat it. Inadequate patient education leads to impaired patient decision making. Patients with DCIS grossly overestimate their risk of recurrence after treatment, the risk of subsequent invasive cancer, and the risk of metastatic spread. For example, even though the actual risk of metastatic spread is close to zero, a 2008 study found that 28 percent of DCIS patients thought this event was "moderately likely."[19] Given these misperceptions and the news that the cancer was caught at the earliest possible stage, some patients take the "I may not be so lucky next time" approach and opt to undergo surgical removal of both breasts.

Finally, the way radiologists view DCIS needs to change. Two factors inform the approach of American radiologists to this condition. These are, first, the deeply held but unproven view that finding DCIS today prevents invasive cancer tomorrow, and second, the ubiquitous threat of malpractice litigation. Our medical training dictates that we assiduously seek out and analyze all potentially suspicious microcalcifications. We are constantly on the lookout for DCIS that is as small as the proverbial "period at the end of this sentence." It has been observed that the rate of DCIS detection in the

United States is higher than in other developed countries with active mammography screening programs. For example, U.S. rates are three times higher than in the United Kingdom.[20] This has been positively correlated with the higher screening recall rates—the proportion of women who receive an abnormal screening mammogram report and are asked to return for additional imaging—in America.[21] The recall rate is a delicate statistic that requires a careful balancing act. A recall rate that is too low, such as 1 or 2 percent, implies that the radiologist may be missing small, subtle cancers, and so the effectiveness of screening may be diminished. If it is too high, say, 20 percent, the overall cost of screening is greatly inflated, usually without any added improvement in its effectiveness. In other words, most of the excess recalls represent false alarms. Radiologists who are inexperienced or who are overly concerned about malpractice litigation often have high recall rates. Recalling a few extra patients may be perceived as a less risky proposition than potentially missing a breast cancer.

The U.S. Agency for Health Care Policy and Research recommends that the screening recall rate be kept below 10 percent.[22] Radiologists in the United Kingdom and the European Union are held to a somewhat more stringent standard of less than 7 percent and less than 5 percent, respectively.[23] Despite the published U.S. guideline of 10 percent, actual clinical results are often far off the mark. One large study that reviewed the results of over 5 million screening mammograms in the United States and the United Kingdom showed a U.S. recall rate of 14.4 percent compared with 7.6 percent in the UK.[24]

Microcalcifications are the second most common reason for recalling women after screening. Typically, magnified mammographic views are performed at the return visit. Standard radiology teaching requires that a biopsy be recommended for all but the most obviously benign-looking microcalcifications. If the radiologist feels that there is more than a 2 percent likelihood of DCIS, the usual practice is to recommend a biopsy, regardless of whether the abnormality is the size of a dot or the size of a dime.

Given what is known about the low biological potential of many mammographically identified DCIS lesions, I believe that radiologists should rethink this aggressive approach to microcalcifications. A more rational approach would involve a reduced role for biopsy, particularly for the tiniest lesions, and an expanded role for short-term follow-up mammography, in which the patient is monitored at six-month intervals. If a particular cluster of microcalcifications does not change over a multiyear follow-up period, one can assume that it represents either something completely benign or DCIS that does not need to be diagnosed. This new approach, in which diagnosing DCIS is deemphasized, would require a radical change in the thinking of the radiology community. It would also require consensus among oncologists, surgeons, and other medical professionals involved in the care of women with breast cancer.

Not only should radiologists' zeal for finding DCIS on mammography be throttled, but also this new thinking needs to extend to other imaging technologies as well. The "Go in Search" dispensation of the past several decades has seen a parade of increasingly sophisticated breast imaging devices. Many of these have been promoted for their superior DCIS-detecting capabilities. Innovations such as computer-aided detection (CAD) and digital mammography both result in higher rates of calcification detection and DCIS diagnoses.[25] In addition, it is now becoming standard practice for women with newly diagnosed breast cancer to undergo magnetic resonance imaging (MRI) of the breasts prior to surgery. The rationale for this approach is that MRI is superior to mammography at finding other, unsuspected tumors in the diseased breast as well as in the opposite breast. In a large study of 969 women with recently diagnosed breast cancer who underwent MRI, thirty were found to have an unsuspected cancer in the opposite breast. In all these patients, mammography had shown nothing suspicious in the opposite breast. Of the thirty unsuspected cancers, twelve were DCIS.[26] Prior to the widespread adoption of MRI for this purpose, these unsuspected tumors, which surely have always existed, would have been adequately controlled by the systemic therapy (chemotherapy or hormonal therapy) the patient received for the *known* cancer. By having them documented preoperatively, however, the patient is obliged to undergo additional surgery. In many cases, out of a combination of fear and exasperation, patients opt to have both breasts removed.

Final Thoughts

Mammography-induced overdiagnosis, particularly of DCIS, is the most significant risk of screening. While the subject is complex, the proponents of screening must do a better job of educating the public about this issue. Women referred for mammography need to know not only that mammography may reduce their risk of dying of breast cancer but also that some mammography-detected cancers would never have caused symptoms in their lifetime. Women diagnosed with DCIS need to be better informed about what is known and what is not known about the natural course of this disease. Radiologists need to rethink the current approach, which emphasizes fishing out every case of DCIS in the biological reservoir by using increasingly sophisticated technology. It is clear that at the present time, our ability to find DCIS far exceeds our understanding of it. Finally, a concerted research effort is needed, the goal of which is to acquire the necessary tools to allow a better-tailored approach to the treatment of patients with DCIS. The ability to separate trivial DCIS cases from potentially more serious ones will reduce the overdiagnosis-overtreatment burden and make mammography a more effective tool.

Despite the myriad controversies in its more than forty-year history, mammography remains an indispensable tool in the fight against breast cancer. Between 1990 and 2007, the U.S. breast cancer death rate decreased by 31 percent, from 33.30 per 100,000 women to 22.91 per 100,000 women.[27] How much of this decline is due to screening and early detection is hotly debated. A 2011 study comparing pairs of European countries that began large-scale mammographic screening many years apart but had similar access to modern therapies found that breast cancer mortality declined to a similar degree.[28] The authors concluded that all of the improvement in breast cancer mortality was attributable to improved therapy and none to screening. An earlier study estimated that almost half (46 percent) of the improvement was due to early detection through screening mammography, with the remainder due to improvements in therapy.[29] The truth likely lies somewhere between these two results.

Screening benefits women aged forty to forty-nine and those who are fifty and older. The magnitude of the benefit, however, is greater for those over fifty. With the battle for access essentially having been won, I believe that mammography should and will continue to be available to all women over forty who wish to be screened.

This battle over access to mammography, spanning the period 1976–2010, was fought and won by the backers of screening, in part by carefully managing the "mammography message." This strategy of consistently promoting the benefits of screening (even at times when the benefits were more *presumed* than *proven*), while remaining largely silent on its potential harms, proved highly successful. Yet it is well known that mammography does have certain risks. Chief among these are the risks of false readings (false positives as well as false negatives) and overdiagnosis. Women of all ages need complete and accurate information regarding the risks and benefits of screening. The pro-screening community should finally free itself from the pervasive fear of discussing the limitations of mammography openly and honestly. Our patients expect it and will thank us for it.

NOTES

1. TIMING IS EVERYTHING

1. Submission of a Resolution Relating to Cancer Research, S. Res. 376, 91st Cong., 2nd sess., *Congressional Record* 116 (March 25, 1970), 9260–61.

2. Lawrence K. Altman, "National Cancer Control Effort Equal to Space Push Is Sought," *New York Times*, November 6, 1969.

3. Submission of a Resolution Relating to Cancer Research, 9262.

4. Additional Statements of Senators, 91st Cong., 2nd sess., *Congressional Record* 116 (July 6, 1970), 22785–86.

5. Bentsen would go on to defeat his Republican opponent, Congressman George H. W. Bush, in the November general election, becoming the junior senator from Texas in the Ninety-second Congress. Bush would again make a cameo appearance in the history of screening mammography twenty years later as the thirty-ninth president.

6. John T. Wooley and Gerhard Peters, "Richard Nixon: Twenty-sixth Annual Message to the Congress on the State of the Union," January 22, 1971, http://www.presidency.ucsb.edu/ws/?pid=3110 (accessed December 3, 2009).

7. John T. Wooley and Gerhard Peters, "Statement about the National Cancer Act of 1971," December 23, 1971, http://www.presidency.ucsb.edu/ws/?pid=3276 (accessed November 25, 2009).

8. National Cancer Institute, "National Cancer Act of 1971," http://www.cancer.gov/aboutnci/national-cancer-act-1971 (accessed February 16, 2010).

9. Carol Weisman, *Women's Health Care: Activist Traditions and Institutional Change* (Baltimore: Johns Hopkins University Press, 1998), 68–69.

10. Ibid., 73.

11. Mary Zimmerman, "The Women's Health Movement: A Critique of Medical Enterprise and the Position of Women," in *Analyzing Gender: A Handbook of Social Science Research*, ed. Beth B. Hess and Myra M. Ferree (Newbury Park, Calif.: Sage, 1987), 443.

12. Sheryl B. Ruzek, *The Women's Health Movement: Feminist Alternatives to Medical Control* (New York: Praeger, 1978), 18.

13. Zimmerman, "Women's Health Movement," 455–61.

14. Boston Women's Health Book Collective, *Our Bodies, Ourselves: A Book by and for Women* (New York: Simon and Schuster, 1971), 1.

15. Ruzek, "Women's Health Movement," 53.

16. Zimmerman, "Women's Health Movement," 456.

17. Weisman, *Women's Health Care*, 75.

18. Ibid., 76.

19. Kirsten E. Gardner, *Early Detection: Women, Cancer, and Awareness Campaigns in the Twentieth-Century United States* (Chapel Hill: University of North Carolina Press, 2006), 208.

20. William S. Halsted, "The Results of Operations for the Cure of Cancer of the Breast Performed at the Johns Hopkins Hospital from June 1889, to January 1894," *Annals of Surgery* 20 (1894): 497–555.

21. Samuel H. Adams, "What Can We Do about Cancer?" *Ladies' Home Journal*, May 1913, 21–22.

22. Gardner, *Early Detection*, 19.

23. Ibid., 74–76.

24. Irvin Fleming, Harmon Eyre, and Jan Pogue, *The American Cancer Society: A History of Saving Lives* (Atlanta: American Cancer Society, 2010), 24.

25. "Medicine: Cancer Army," Time.com, March 22, 1937, http://www.time.com/time/magazine/article/0,9171,757452,00.html (accessed January 7, 2010).

26. Gardner, *Early Detection*, 77.

27. Ibid., 103–4.

28. Ibid., 110–11.

29. Fleming, Eyre, and Pogue, *American Cancer Society*, 48–49.

30. Gardner, *Early Detection*, 104–5.

31. Ibid., 105.

32. George N. Papanicolaou, "New Cancer Diagnosis," *CA: A Cancer Journal for Clinicians* 23 (1973): 174–79.

33. Practically across the street from ACS headquarters. This geographic proximity played a role in the organization's learning about Papanicolaou's work.

34. An open biopsy is a surgical operation where a biopsy is performed.

35. Cyrus C. Erickson, "Exfoliative Cytology in Mass Screening for Uterine Cancer: Memphis and Shelby County, Tennessee," *CA: A Cancer Journal for Clinicians* 5 (1955): 63–64.

36. Ibid.

37. Raymond F. Kaiser and Cyrus C. Erickson, "Initial Effect of Community-Wide Cytologic Screening on Clinical Stage of Cervical Cancer Detected in an Entire Community: Results of Memphis–Shelby County, Tennessee, Study," *Journal of the National Cancer Institute* 25 (1960): 863.

38. Fleming, Eyre, and Pogue, *American Cancer Society*, 63–64.

39. American Cancer Society, "Statistics on Cancer," *CA: A Cancer Journal for Clinicians* 18 (1968): 18.

2. FIRST EXPOSURE

1. Bruce J. Hillman, "The Diffusion of New Imaging Technologies: A Molecular Imaging Prospective," *Journal of the American College of Radiology* 3 (2006): 34.

2. National Cancer Institute, "5-year Cancer Mortality Rates per 100,000 Person-Years, Age-Adjusted 1970 U.S. Population. Breast 1950–1994, All Ages," http://www3.cancer.gov/atlasplus/ (accessed February 16, 2010); Barron H. Lerner, *The Breast Cancer Wars: Fear, Hope, and the Pursuit of a Cure in Twentieth-Century America* (New York: Oxford University Press, 2001), 202

3. Stafford Warren, "A Roentgenologic Study of the Breast," *American Journal of Roentgenology and Radium Therapy* 24 (1930): 113–24.

4. J. Gershon-Cohen, M. B. Hermel, and S. M. Berger, "Detection of Breast Cancer by Periodic X-Ray Examinations," *Journal of the American Medical Association* 176 (1961): 1114–16.

5. Robert L. Egan, "Experience with Mammography in a Tumor Institution: Evaluation of 1,000 Studies," *Radiology* 75 (1960): 895.

6. Bettyann Holtzmann Kevles, *Naked to the Bone: Medical Imaging in the Twentieth Century* (New Brunswick, N.J.: Rutgers University Press, 1997), 253.

7. R. Lee Clark, Murray M. Copeland, and Robert L. Egan, "Reproducibility of the Technic of Mammography (Egan) for Cancer of the Breast," *American Journal of Surgery* 109 (1965): 127–33.

8. Arthur I. Holleb, "Review of Breast Cancer Screening Guidelines," *Cancer* 69 (1992): 1911–12.

9. Sam Shapiro, Wanda Venet, Philip Strax, and Louis Venet, *Periodic Screening for Breast Cancer: The Health Insurance Plan Project and Its Sequelae, 1963–1986* (Baltimore: Johns Hopkins University Press, 1988), 10–11.

10. Sam Shapiro, Philip Strax, and Louis Venet, "Periodic Breast Cancer Screening in Reducing Mortality from Breast Cancer," *Journal of the American Medical Association* 215 (1971): 1777–85.

11. Jane E. Brody, "Cancer Studies Back Screening," *New York Times*, May 19, 1971.

12. Holleb, "Review of Breast Cancer Screening."

13. Oliver H. Beahrs, Sam Shapiro, and Charles Smart, "Report of the Working Group to Review the National Cancer Institute–American Cancer Society Breast Cancer Detection Demonstration Projects," *Journal of the National Cancer Institute* 62 (1979): 651.

14. Thermography was ultimately discontinued in the program's second year owing to a lack of effectiveness in finding early stage breast cancer.

15. Holleb, "Review of Breast Cancer Screening."

16. Lerner, *Breast Cancer Wars*, 206.

17. Maren Klawiter, *The Biopolitics of Breast Cancer: Changing Cultures of Disease and Activism* (Minneapolis: University of Minnesota Press, 2008), 89.

18. Lerner, *Breast Cancer Wars*, 206.

19. American Cancer Society News Service, press release, January 8, 1973.

20. Daniel Greenberg, "X-Ray Mammography: Background to a Decision," *New England Journal of Medicine* 295 (September 1976): 739–40.

21. Holleb, "Review of Breast Cancer Screening," 1911.

22. American Cancer Society News Service, press release, January 8, 1973; American Cancer Society News Service, press release, February 8, 1974.

23. Benjamin F. Byrd and William H. Hartmann, "Breast Cancer Detection Epoch," *Seminars in Surgical Oncology* 4 (1988): 222.

24. Larry H. Baker, "Breast Cancer Detection Demonstration Project: Five-Year Summary Report," *CA: A Cancer Journal for Clinicians* 32 (1982): 196.

25. American Cancer Society, "Finding Breast Cancer Before It Can Be Felt," *Cancer News* (Spring–Summer 1974): 14.

26. John T. Wooley and Gerhard Peters, "Gerald Ford: Remarks Concluding the Summit Conference on Inflation September 28, 1974," http://www.presidency.ucsb.edu/ws/?pid=4420 (accessed December 3, 2009).

27. David A. Andelman, "Wife of Rockefeller Has Breast Cancer Operation," *New York Times*, October 18, 1974.

28. Ibid.

29. John Stowell, "Women Cautioned on Breast X-Rays," *Washington Post*, April 25, 1975.

30. Beahrs, Shapiro, and Smart, "Report of the Working Group," 663.

31. L. K. Altman, "Swine Flu Program Suspended in Nation: Disease Link Feared," *New York Times*, December 17, 1976.

32. U.S. Department of Health, Education and Welfare, "Background Statement: NIH/ACS Consensus Development Meeting on Breast Cancer Screening" (Bethesda, Md.: U.S. Department of Health, Education and Welfare, National Institutes of Health, 1977).

33. Stuart Auerbach, "Breast X-Ray Backed," *Washington Post*, November 7, 1975.

34. Irvin Fleming, Harmon Eyre, and Jan Pogue, *The American Cancer Society: A History of Saving Lives* (Atlanta: American Cancer Society, 2010), 183–85.

35. John C. Bailar, "Mammography: A Contrary View," *Annals of Internal Medicine* 84 (1976): 77–84.

36. Ibid.

37. Daniel S. Greenberg and Judith E. Randal, "The Questionable Breast X-Ray Program," *Washington Post,* May 1, 1977.

38. "Breast X-Ray Form to Contain Warning," *Washington Post,* March 27, 1976.

39. U.S. Department of Health, Education and Welfare, "Statement on X-Ray Mammography in Screening for Breast Cancer" (Bethesda, Md.: U.S. Department of Health, Education and Welfare, National Institutes of Health, 1976), 2.

40. Victor Cohn, "Women Avoiding Breast Cancer Test," *Washington Post,* November 23, 1976.

41. Ibid.

42. Walter S. Ross, "What Every Woman Should Know about Breast X-Ray," *Reader's Digest,* March 1977, 118–19.

43. Genell Subak-Sharpe, "Is Mammography Safe? Yes, No and Maybe," *New York Times,* October 24, 1976.

44. Jerry D. Boyd, ed., "Mammography Guidelines Tightened, Limited to High Risk Groups," *Cancer Letter,* May 13, 1977, 4–5.

45. Beahrs, Shapiro, and Smart, "Report of the Working Group," 650.

46. Randy Shilts, *And the Band Played On: Politics, People, and the AIDS Epidemic* (New York: St. Martin's Press, 1987), 141–42.

3. THE AFTERMATH

1. Larry H. Baker, "Breast Cancer Detection Demonstration Project: Five-Year Summary Report," *CA: A Cancer Journal for Clinicians* 32 (1982): 194–225.

2. Maren Klawiter, *The Biopolitics of Breast Cancer: Changing Cultures of Disease and Activism* (Minneapolis: University of Minnesota Press, 2008), 86, 102.

3. Ibid., 95.

4. Ibid.

5. Ibid.

6. Danzu Rosner, Ramez N. Bedwani, Josef Vana, Harvey W. Baker, and Gerald P. Murphy, "Noninvasive Breast Carcinoma: Results of a National Survey by the American College of Surgeons," *Annals of Surgery* 192 (1980): 139.

7. Charles R. Smart, Celia Byrne, Robert A. Smith, Lawrence Garfinkel, A. Hamblin Letton, Gerald D. Dodd, and Oliver H. Beahrs, "Twenty-Year Follow-up of the Breast Cancers Diagnosed during the Breast Cancer Detection Demonstration Project," *CA: A Cancer Journal for Clinicians* 47 (1997): 139.

8. Christopher I. Li, Janet R. Daling, and Kathleen E. Malone, "Age-Specific Incidence Rates of in Situ Breast Carcinomas by Histologic Type, 1980–2001," *Cancer Epidemiology, Biomarkers, and Prevention* 14 (2005): 1009.

9. Karla Kerlikowske, "Epidemiology of Ductal Carcinoma in Situ," in *NIH State-of-the-Science Conference: Diagnosis and Management of Ductal Carcinoma in Situ (DCIS)* (Bethesda, Md.: U.S. Department of Health and Human Services, National Institutes of Health, 2009), 25.

10. Melinda E. Sanders, Peggy A. Schuyler, William D. Dupont, and David L. Page, "The Natural History of Low-Grade Ductal Carcinoma in Situ of the Breast in Women Treated by Biopsy Only Revealed over 30 Years of Long-Term Follow-Up," *Cancer* 103 (2005): 2481.

11. H. Gilbert Welch and William C. Black, "Overdiagnosis in Cancer," *Journal of the National Cancer Institute* 102 (2010): 605–13.

12. American Cancer Society, "Cancer Facts and Figures, 2009" (Atlanta: American Cancer Society, 2009).

13. American Cancer Society, "Mammography Guidelines, 1983: Background Statement and Update of Cancer-Related Checkup; Guidelines for Breast Cancer Detection in Asymptomatic Women Age 40–49," *CA: A Cancer Journal for Clinicians* 33 (1983): 255.

14. Victor Cohn, "Cancer Group Prescribes Breast X-Rays after 40," *Washington Post*, August 3, 1983.

15. Gerald D. Dodd, "American College of Radiology Commission on Cancer: Interim Statement on Breast Cancer Diagnosis," *Journal of the Tennessee Medical Association* 69 (1976): 640–41.

16. Ibid., 640; emphasis added.

17. American College of Radiology, "New ACR Guidelines on Mammography," *ACR Bulletin* (November 1982): 6–7.

18. Kenneth C. Chu, Charles R. Smart, and Robert E. Tarone, "Analysis of Breast Cancer Mortality and Stage Distribution by Age for the Health Insurance Plan Clinical Trial," *Journal of the National Cancer Institute* 80 (1988): 1125–32.

19. Cori Vanchieri, "Breast Cancer Screening: Evidence of Benefit for Women 40–49," *Journal of the National Cancer Institute* 80 (1988): 1090–92.

20. The organizations included in the Medical Roundtable were the American Medical Association, National Cancer Institute, American Academy of Family Physicians, American Association of Women Radiologists, American Osteopathic College of Radiology, American Society of Therapeutic Radiology and Oncology, American Society of Internal Medicine, College of American Pathologists, National Medical Association, American Cancer Society, and American College of Radiology.

21. Cori Vanchieri, "Medical Groups Message to Women: If 40 or Older, Get Regular Mammograms," *Journal of the National Cancer Institute* 81 (1989): 1126–28.

22. U.S. Preventive Services Task Force, *Guide to Clinical Preventive Services: An Assessment of the Effectiveness of 169 Interventions* (Baltimore: William and Wilkins, 1989), 39–46.

23. American College of Physicians, "The Use of Diagnostic Tests for Screening and Evaluating Breast Lesions," *Annals of Internal Medicine* 103 (1985): 143–46.

4. A TALE OF TWO EPIDEMICS

1. M. S. Gottlieb, H. M. Schanker, P. T. Fran, A. Saxon, and J. D. Weisman, "Pneumocystis Pneumonia—Los Angeles," *MMWR: Morbidity and Mortality Weekly Report* 30 (1981): 1–3.

2. U.S. Centers for Disease Control, "Current Trends: Update on Acquired Immune Deficiency Syndrome (AIDS)—United States," *MMWR: Morbidity and Mortality Weekly Reports* 31 (1982): 507–8.

3. U.S. Centers for Disease Control, "Current Trends Update: Acquired Immunodeficiency Syndrome (AIDS)—United States," *MMWR: Morbidity and Mortality Weekly Reports* 32 (1983): 465–67.

4. Randy Shilts, *And the Band Played On: Politics, People, and the AIDS Epidemic* (New York: St. Martin's Press, 1987), xxii.

5. John T. Wooley and Gerhard Peters, "Ronald Reagan: Remarks at the American Foundation for AIDS Research Awards Dinner," American Presidency Project, May 31, 1987, http://www.presidency.ucsb.edu/ws/?pid=34348 (accessed June 8, 2010).

6. Shilts, *And the Band Played On*, xxii.

7. Deborah Gould, *Moving Politics: Emotion and ACT UP's Fight against AIDS* (Chicago: University of Chicago Press, 2009), 75.

8. Dennis Altman, *AIDS in the Mind of America: The Social, Political, and Psychological Impact of a New Epidemic* (Garden City, N.Y.: Anchor Books, 1987), 109.

9. Gould, *Moving Politics*, 89–90.

10. Ibid., 65.

11. Shilts, *And the Band Played On*, 122.

12. Gould, *Moving Politics*, 92–93.

13. Altman, *AIDS in the Mind of America*, 107.

14. Tony Mauro, *Illustrated Great Decisions of the Supreme Court* (Washington, D.C.: CQ Press, 2000), 14–17.

15. U.S. Centers for Disease Control, "Current Trends Update: Acquired Immunodeficiency Syndrome—United States," *MMWR: Morbidity and Mortality Weekly Report* 35 (1986): 757–60, 765–66.

16. Gould, *Moving Politics*, 122–32.

17. Steven Epstein, *Impure Science: AIDS, Activism, and the Politics of Knowledge* (Berkeley: University of California Press, 1996), 219–26.

18. Karlyn Barker and Linda Wheeler, "Hundreds of Thousands March for Gay Rights: People from Across U.S. Converge on Mall," *Washington Post*, October 12, 1987.

19. Irvin Molotsky, "Congress Passes Compromise AIDS Bill," *New York Times*, October 14, 1988.

20. Warren E. Leary, "FDA Announces Changes to Speed Testing of Drugs," *New York Times*, October 20, 1988.

21. Epstein, *Impure Science,* 219–26.

22. Ted Kreiter and Cory SerVaas, "Chasing Cancer with Sonar," *Saturday Evening Post*, September 1980, 26–31; Lane Lenard, "Breast Cancer: New Ways to Spot It Early," *McCalls*, November 1984, 44.

23. American Cancer Society, "1989 Survey of Physicians' Attitudes and Practices in Early Detection," *CA: A Cancer Journal for Clinicians* 40 (1990): 81.

24. Tom Morganthau, Thomas DeFrank, and Mary Hager, "Let's Just Hold Hands," *Newsweek*, October 26, 1987, 28–29; Lawrence K. Altman, "Surgeons Remove Cancerous Breast of Nancy Reagan," *New York Times*, October 17, 1987.

25. "More Women Seek X-Rays of Breasts," *New York Times*, November 1, 1987.

26. Herbert Seidman, Margaret H. Mushinski, Steven K. Gelb, and Edwin Silverberg, "Probabilities of Eventually Developing or Dying of Cancer—United States, 1985," *CA: A Cancer Journal for Clinicians* 35 (1985): 36–56; Herbert Seidman, Edwin Silverberg, and Ashley Bodden, "Probabilities of Eventually Developing and Dying of Cancer," *CA: A Cancer Journal for Clinicians* 28 (1978): 33–46.

27. Ruth Spear, "Breast Cancer: New Facts, New Fears," *Ladies' Home Journal*, February 1988, 71–74; Leslie Laurence, "The Breast Cancer Epidemic: Women Aren't Just Scared, We're Mad," *McCalls*, November 1991, 24–40.

28. Melinda Beck, Emily Yoffe, Ginny Carroll, Mary Hager, Debra Rosenberg, and Lucille Beachy, "The Politics of Breast Cancer," *Newsweek*, December 10, 1990, 63.

29. Steven Dickman, "Fighting for Their Lives," *U.S. News and World Report*, August 26, 1991, 70.

30. Ibid.

31. Beck et al., "Politics of Breast Cancer," 62–63.

32. Ibid., 63.

33. U.S. Centers for Disease Control, "Use of Mammography—United States, 1990," *MMWR: Morbidity and Mortality Weekly Reports* 39 (1990): 621.

34. Molly Sinclair, "Cancer Measures Signed," *Washington Post*, May 22, 1986.

35. Beck et al., "Politics of Breast Cancer," 63.

36. "Stat Bite: State Mammography Legislation," *Journal of the National Cancer Institute* 85 (1993): 605.

37. Paul Goldberg and Jerry Boyd, "Medicare to Pay for Mammography, Defines 'Covered Drugs' Broadly," *Cancer Economics*, June 24, 1988, 1, 5.

38. Spencer Rich, "Catastrophic Health Law Is Repealed by Congress: Effort to Save Some Benefits Is Swept Aside," *Washington Post*, November 22, 1989.

39. U.S. Centers for Disease Control, "National Breast and Cervical Cancer Early Detection Program, July 1991–July 1992," *MMWR: Morbidity and Mortality Weekly Report* 41 (October 9, 1992), 739–43.

40. Eliot Marshall, "The Politics of Breast Cancer," *Science* 259 (January 1993): 616–17.

41. Neil Lewis, "Law Professor Accuses Thomas of Sexual Harassment in 1980s," *New York Times*, October 7, 1991.

42. R. W. Apple, "The 1992 Elections: President Elect—The Overview; Clinton, Savoring Victory, Starts Sizing Up Job Ahead," *New York Times*, November 5, 1992.

43. Carol S. Weisman, "Breast Cancer Policymaking," in *Breast Cancer: Society Shapes an Epidemic*, ed. Anne Kasper and Susan J. Ferguson (New York: Palgrave, 2000), 216.

44. Martin L. Brown, Larry G. Kessler, and Fred G. Reuter, "Is the Oversupply of Mammography Machines Outstripping Need and Demand?" *Annals of Internal Medicine* 113 (1990): 548–49; Burton J. Conway, John L. McCrohan, Fred G. Rueter, and Orhan H. Suleiman, "Mammography in the Eighties," *Radiology* 177 (1990): 335; Florence Houn and Martin L. Brown, "Current Practice of Screening Mammography in the United States: Data from the National Survey of Mammography Facilities," *Radiology* 190 (1994): 210.

45. Conway et al., "Mammography in the Eighties," 337.

46. Jerry D. Boyd, ed., "More Than 450 Mammography Facilities Are Accredited by the American College of Radiology," *Cancer Letter*, April 7, 1989, 1–4; "At Least One Mammography Unit in Every State Is Accredited," *Cancer Letter*, May 18, 1990, 5–7.

47. Michele Gillen, "Medicine: Breast Cancer" (pts. 1, 2, and 3), *NBC Nightly News*, June 20–22, 1990.

48. Eric Feuer, Lap-Ming Wun, Catherine Boring, W. Dana Flanders, Marilyn Timmel, and Tony Tong, "The Lifetime Risk of Developing Breast Cancer," *Journal of the National Cancer Institute* 85 (1993): 892–97.

49. Sandra Blakeslee, "Better Odds: Faulty Math Heightens Fears of Breast Cancer," *New York Times*, March 15, 1992; emphasis added.

50. Karen M. Kedrowski and Marilyn S. Sarrow, *Cancer Activism: Gender, Media, and Public Policy* (Urbana: University of Illinois Press, 2007), 94–97.

5. AGE IS NOTHING BUT A NUMBER

1. John Cassidy and Tim Rayment, "Breast Scans Boost Risk of Cancer Death," *Sunday Times* (London), June 2, 1991.

2. A companion study, the CNBSS-2, found that annual mammography plus physical examination did not reduce mortality in women fifty and older compared to physical examination alone.

3. Anthony B. Miller, Cornelia J. Baines, Teresa To, and Claus Wall, "Canadian National Breast Screening Study: 1. Breast Cancer Detection and Death Rates among Women Aged 40–49 Years," *Canadian Medical Association Journal* 147 (1992): 1459–60.

4. American College of Radiology, "ACR Criticizes Mammography Study," *ACR Bulletin* 48 (December 1992): 7.

5. A "statistically significant" result is one that is strong enough to be considered scientifically reliable. A result that is not statistically significant could possibly be caused by chance and so is not reliable.

6. There were actually seven speakers on the first day of the conference. The seventh, however, R. E. Hendrick, a medical physicist, discussed technical quality issues in mammography. Walter Lawrence and Robert Smith, "Conference Summary," *Cancer* 72, supplement 4 (1993): 1491–95.

7. Curtis J. Mettlin and Charles R. Smart, "The Canadian National Breast Screening Study: An Appraisal and Implications for Early Detection Policy," *Cancer* 72, supplement 4 (1993): 1461–65.

8. S. W. Fletcher and R. H. Fletcher, "The Breast Is Close to the Heart," *Annals of Internal Medicine* 117 (1992): 970.

9. Suzanne W. Fletcher, William Black, Russell Harris, Barbara K. Rimer, and Sam Shapiro, "Report of the International Workshop on Screening for Breast Cancer," *Journal of the National Cancer Institute* 85 (1993): 1644.

10. Opponents of under-fifty screening contend that age fifty is an important benchmark because it is close to the average age of menopause for American women.

11. Daniel Kopans, "Controversy: Mammography Screening of Women Aged 40–49," *SBI News* (March 1994): 2.

12. Charles Marwick, "NCI Board Votes to Keep Mammography Guidelines," *Journal of the American Medical Association* 270 (1993): 2783.

13. Nancy Volkers, "Expert Board Gives Advice to NCI on Breast Cancer Screening Guidelines," *Journal of the National Cancer Institute* 85 (1993): 1795.

14. Marwick, "NCI Board Votes," 2783.

15. Bernadine Healy, "Pricing Health Care: Mammograms—Your Breasts, Your Choice," *Wall Street Journal*, December 28, 1993.

16. "Expressing the Sense of the House of Representatives with Respect to the Inclusion in Any Comprehensive Benefits Package under Health Care Reform of Mammography Screenings for Women under the Age of 50," H. R. Res. 368, 103rd Cong., 2nd sess. *Congressional Record* 140 (February 23, 1994), H 566.

17. House of Representatives, Human Resources and Intergovernmental Relations Subcommittee of the Committee on Government Operations, 103rd Cong., 2nd sess., *National Cancer Institute's Revision of Its Mammography Guidelines* (Washington, D.C.: U.S. Government Printing Office, 1994).

18. House of Representatives, Human Resources and Intergovernmental Relations Subcommittee of the Committee on Government Operations, 103rd Cong., 2nd sess., *Misused Science: The National Cancer Institute's Elimination of Mammography Guidelines for Women in Their Forties* (Washington, D.C.: U.S. Government Printing Office, 1994).

19. Ibid., 13.

20. Senate Subcommittee on Departments of Labor, Health and Human Services, and Education, and Related Agencies, 105 Cong., 1st sess., *Mammography: Hearings before a Subcommittee of the Committee on Appropriations* (Washington, D.C.: U.S. Government Printing Office, 1997), 3.

21. Organizing Committee and Collaborators, Falun Meeting, Falun, Sweden, March 21–22, 1996, "Breast Cancer Screening with Mammography in Women Aged 40–49 Years," *International Journal of Cancer* 68 (1996): 693–99.

22. House of Representatives, Human Resources and Intergovernmental Relations Subcommittee of the Committee on Government Operations, *National Cancer Institute's Revision of Its Mammography Guidelines*, 1.

23. One panel member resigned in protest prior to publication of the conference report.

24. R. Edward Hendrick, "Update of the NIH Consensus Development Conference on Breast Cancer Screening for Women Ages 40–49," *SBI News* (February 1997): 5.

25. National Institutes of Health Consensus Development Panel, "National Institutes of Health Consensus Development Conference Statement: Breast Cancer Screening for Women Ages 40–49, January 21–23, 1997," *Journal of the National Cancer Institute* 14 (1997): 1019.

26. Gina Kolata, "Stand on Mammograms Greeted by Outrage," *New York Times*, January 28, 1997.

27. Gina Kolata, "Mammogram Talks Prove Indefinite," *New York Times*, January 24, 1997.

28. Ibid.

29. Bernadine P. Healy, "Screening Mammography for Women in Their Forties: The Panel of Babel," *Journal of Women's Health* 6 (1997): 1.

30. Senate Subcommittee on Departments of Labor, Health and Human Services, and Education, and Related Agencies, *Mammography*, 73–74.

31. National Institutes of Health Consensus Development Panel, "National Institutes of Health Consensus Development Conference Statement," 1015.

32. Senate Subcommittee on Departments of Labor, Health and Human Services, and Education, and Related Agencies, *Mammography*, 72–73.

33. Ibid., 2.

34. Carol S. Weisman, "Breast Cancer Policymaking," in *Breast Cancer: Society Shapes an Epidemic*, ed. Anne Kasper and Susan J. Ferguson (New York: Palgrave, 2000), 216.

35. Senate Subcommittee on Departments of Labor, Health and Human Services, and Education, and Related Agencies, *Mammography*, 198.

36. David Brown, "Mammogram Test Advice Stirs Debate: Cancer Group Urges Yearly Exam in 40s," *Washington Post*, March 24, 1997.

37. Peggy Eastman, "NCI Adopts New Mammography Screening Guidelines for Women," *Journal of the National Cancer Institute* 8 (1997): 538.

6. PULLING THE PLUG ON GRANNY

1. Gina Kolata, "Cancer Group Has Concerns on Screening," *New York Times*, October 21, 2009.

2. Laura Esserman, Yiwey Shieh, and Ian Thompson, "Rethinking Screening for Breast Cancer and Prostate Cancer," *Journal of the American Medical Association* 302 (2009): 1685–92.

3. U.S. Preventive Services Task Force, "Screening for Breast Cancer: U.S. Preventive Services Task Force Recommendation Statement," *Annals of Internal Medicine* 151 (2009): 716.

4. Ibid.

5. Rob Stein and Dan Eggen, "White House Backs Off Cancer Test Guidelines," *Washington Post*, November 19, 2009.

6. American College of Radiology, "USPSTF Mammography Recommendations Will Result in Countless Unnecessary Breast Cancer Deaths Each Year," November 16, 2009, http://www.acr.org/MainMenuCategories/media_room/FeaturedCategories/PressReleases/USPSTFMammoRecs.aspx (accessed February 20, 2010).

7. Stein and Eggen, "White House Backs Off."

8. Otis Brawley, "Let's Stick with Mammograms," *Washington Post*, November 19, 2009.

9. Daniel Kopans, interviewed by Campbell Brown on *Campbell Brown: No Bias, No Bull*, CNN, November 18, 2009.

10. Gina Kolata, "Mammogram Debate Took Group by Surprise," *New York Times*, November 20, 2009.

11. Jane Norman, "Brinker Cites 'Justifiable Outrage' on Mammography Recommendations," *CQ HealthBeat*, November 23, 2009, http://global.factiva.com (accessed November 4, 2011).

12. House of Representatives, Health Subcommittee of the House Energy and Commerce Committee, "Hearing of the Health Subcommittee of the House Energy and Commerce Committee (Part 27)," Federal News Service, December 3, 2009, http://global.factiva.com (accessed February 21, 2011).

13. Susan Love, interviewed by Robin Roberts, "Breast Cancer Screening: When Should Women Start?" *Good Morning America*, ABC News, November 17, 2009.

14. Susan Love, "A Message from Dr. Love about the New Mammography Guidelines," Dr. Susan Love Research Foundation, November 18, 2009, http://blog.dslrf.org/?m=200911 (accessed February 24, 2011).

15. Ibid.

16. Lydia Saad, "Women Disagree with New Mammography Advice," November 24, 2009, http://www.gallup.com/poll/124463/women-disagree-new-mammogram-advice.aspx (accessed February 24, 2011).

17. "Secretary Sebelius Statement on New Breast Cancer Recommendations," U.S. Fed News, November 30, 2009, http://global.factiva.com (accessed February 21, 2011).

18. "Expressing the Sense of the House of Representatives Regarding Guidelines for Breast Cancer Screening for Women Ages 40–49," H.R. Res. 971, 111th Cong., 1st sess. *Congressional Record* 155 (December 15, 2009), H 14910–14916.

19. House of Representatives, Health Subcommittee of the House Energy and Commerce Committee, "Hearing."

20. "Service Members Home Ownership Tax Act of 2009," 111th Cong., 1st sess., *Congressional Record* 155 (December 3, 2009): S12265–S12277.

21. U.S. Department of Health and Human Services, "Administration Announces Regulations Requiring Insurance Plans to Provide Free Preventive Care," July 14, 2010, http://www.hhs.gov/news/press/2010pres/07/20100714a.html (accessed February 20, 2011).

22. John T. Wooley and Gerhard Peters, "Proclamation 8572: National Breast Cancer Awareness Month, 2010," American Presidency Project, October 1, 2010, http://www.presidency.ucsb.edu/ws/?pid=88534 (accessed February 27, 2011).

7. THE HOUSE THAT MAMMOGRAPHY BUILT

1. L. C. Richardson, S. H. Rim, and M. Plescia, "Vital Signs: Breast Cancer Screening among Women Aged 50–74 Years—United States, 2008," *Morbidity and Mortality Weekly Report* 59 (July 2010): 813; Debra L. Blackwell, Michael E. Martinez, and Jane F. Gentleman, "Women's Compliance with Public Health Guidelines for Mammograms and PAP Tests in Canada and the United States: An Analysis of Data from the Joint Canada/United States Survey of Health," *Women's Health Issues* 18 (2008): 90.

2. Physician Insurers Association of America, *Breast Cancer Study*, 3rd ed. (Rockville, Md.: Physician Insurers Association of America, 2002), 9.

3. Karen M. Kedrowski and Marilyn Stine Sarow, *Cancer Activism: Gender, Media, and Public Policy* (Urbana and Chicago: University of Illinois Press, 2007), 97–102.

4. William C. Black, Robert F. Nease, and Anna N. Tosteson, "Perceptions of Breast Cancer Risk and Screening Effectiveness in Women Younger Than 50 Years of Age," *Journal of the National Cancer Institute* 87 (1995): 720–31.

5. Gianfranco Domenighetti, Barbara D'Avanzo, Matthias Egger, Franco Berrino, Thomas Perneger, Paola Mosconi, and Marcel Zwahlen, "Women's Perception of the Benefits of Mammography Screening: Population-Based Survey in Four Countries," *International Journal of Epidemiology* 32 (2003): 818.

6. Ibid.

7. Physician Insurers Association, *Breast Cancer Study*, 2–6.

8. Patricia A. Kaufert, "Women and the Debate over Mammography: An Economic, Political, and Moral History," in *Gender and Health: An International Perspective*, ed. Carolyn F. Sargent and Caroline B. Brettell (Upper Saddle River, N.J.: Prentice Hall, 1996), 175.

9. Rebecca Smith-Bindman, Philip W. Chu, Diana L. Miglioretti, Edward A. Sickles, Roger Blanks, Rachel Ballard-Barbash, Janet K. Bobo, Nancy C. Lee, Matthew G. Wallis, Julietta Patnick, and Karla Kerlikowski, "Comparison of Screening Mammography in the United States and the United Kingdom," *Journal of the American Medical Association* 290 (2003): 2129.

10. Rebecca A. Hubbard, Karla Kerlikowske, Chris I. Flowers, Bonnie C. Yankaskas, Weiwei Zhu, and Diana L. Miglioretti, "Cumulative Probability of False-Positive Recall or Biopsy Recommendation After 10 Years of Screening Mammography," *Annals of Internal Medicine* 155 (2011): 481.

11. Ibid.; Steven P. Poplack, Patricia A. Carney, Julia E. Weiss, Linda Titus-Ernstoff, Martha E. Goodrich, and Anna N. A. Tosteson, "Screening Mammography: Costs and Use of Screening-Related Services," *Radiology* 234 (2005): 79–85.

12. David W. Lee, Paul E. Stang, George A. Goldberg, and Merle Haberman, "Resource Use and Cost of Diagnostic Workup of Women with Suspected Breast Cancer," *Breast Journal* 15 (2009): 85.

13. Lisa M. Schwartz, Steven Woloshin, Floyd J. Fowler Jr., and H. Gilbert Welch, "Enthusiasm for Cancer Screening in the United States," *Journal of the American Medical Association* 291 (2004): 74.

14. Ibid., 74–75.

15. Ibid., 76.

16. Ibid.

17. Lisa M. Schwartz, Steven Woloshin, Harold C. Sox, Baruch Fischhoff, and H. Gilbert Welch, "US Women's Attitudes to False-Positive Mammography Results and Detection of Ductal Carcinoma In Situ: Cross-Sectional Survey," *British Medical Journal* 320 (2000): 1635.

18. Joshua J. Fenton, Linn Abraham, Stephen H. Taplin, Berta M. Geller, Patricia A. Carney, Carl D'Orsi, JoAnn G. Elmore, and William E. Barlow, "Effectiveness of Computer-Aided Detection in Community Mammography Practice," *Journal of the National Cancer Institute* 103 (2011): 1152–61.

19. Wendie A. Berg, Jeffrey D. Blume, Jean B. Cormack, Ellen B. Mendelson, Daniel Lehrer, Marcela Böhm-Vélez, Etta D. Pisano, Roberta A. Jong, W. Phil Evans, Marilyn J. Morton, Mary C. Mahoney, Linda Hovanessian, Richard G. Barr, Dione M. Farria, Helga S. Marques, and Karen Boparai, "Combined Screening with Ultrasound and Mammography Compared to Mammography Alone in Women at Elevated Risk of Breast Cancer: Results of the First-Year Screen in ACRIN 6666," *Journal of the American Medical Association* 299 (2008): 2151.

20. Debbie Saslow, Carla Boetes, Wylie Burke, Steven Harms, Martin O. Leach, Constance D. Lehman, Elizabeth Morris, Etta Pisano, Mitchell Schnall, Stephen Sener, Robert A. Smith, Ellen Warner, Martin Yaffe, Kimberly S. Andrews, and Christy A. Russell, "American Cancer Society Guidelines for Breast Screening with MRI as an Adjunct to Mammography," *CA: A Cancer Journal for Clinicians* 57 (2007): 75.

21. Nancy M. Cappello, areyoudense.org, http://www.areyoudense.org (accessed March 7, 2011).

22. State of Connecticut, Senate Bill no. 422, Public Act no. 06–38, An Act Concerning Health Insurance Coverage for Breast Cancer Screening (May 8, 2006), http://www.cga.ct.gov/2006/ACT/PA/2006PA-00038-R00SB-00422-PA.htm (accessed March 7, 2011).

23. Ibid.

24. "Texas Dense Breast Law Passes," *Cancer Weekly*, July 5, 2011: 114.

25. Steven Harmon, "Brown Weighs in on 200 Bills; Governor OKs Health Care Coverage for Autistic Children, Bans Tanning Beds for Teens," *San Jose Mercury News*, October 10, 2011: 1B.

26. Nancy M. Cappello, "Dense Breast Tissue Awareness," February 3, 2011, http://www.dbtawareness.blogspot.com/2011/02/personal-story-dr-m-cappellodr.html (accessed March 7, 2011).

27. Robert Langreth, "Too Many Mammograms," Forbes.com, November 16, 2009, http://www.forbes.com/2009/11/16/mammograms-cancer-screening-business-healthcare-mammogram.html (accessed March 10, 2011).

28. William E. Barlow, Emily White, Rachel Ballard-Barbash, Pamela M. Vacek, Linda Titus-Ernstoff, Patricia A. Carney, Jeffrey A. Tice, Diana S. M. Buist, Berta M. Geller, Robert Rosenberg, Bonnie C. Yankaskas, and Karla Kerlikowske, "Prospective Breast Cancer Risk Prediction Model for Women Undergoing Screening Mammography," *Journal of the National Cancer Institute* 98 (2006): 1208. Results not directly presented by authors but derived from data in Table 2 (cases with unknown breast density excluded).

29. Melinda E. Sanders, Peggy A. Schuyler, William D. Dupont, and David L. Page, "The Natural History of Low-Grade Ductal Carcinoma In Situ of the Breast in Women Treated by Biopsy Only Revealed over 30 Years of Long-Term Follow-Up," *Cancer* 103 (2005): 2481

30. Cone LLC, "Past, Present, Future: The 25th Anniversary of Cause Marketing" (Boston: Cone LLC, 2008), http://www.coneinc.com (accessed August 23, 2011).

31. DoWellDoGood LLC, "The Do Well Do Good Public Opinion Survey on Cause-Marketing: Summary Report" (Chicago: Do Well Do Good LLC, 2010), http://dowelldogood.net (accessed August 23, 2011).

32. Nancy G. Brinker and Joni Rodgers, *Promise Me: How a Sister's Love Launched the Global Movement to End Breast Cancer* (New York: Crown Archetype, 2010), 258.

33. "Impact of a Promise: 2008–2009 Annual Report, Susan G. Komen for the Cure," Susan G. Komen for the Cure, http://www.komen.org (accessed April 2, 2011).

34. Ibid.

8. OVERDIAGNOSIS: MAMMOGRAPHY'S BURDEN

1. Maren Klawiter, *The Biopolitics of Breast Cancer: Changing Cultures of Disease and Activism* (Minneapolis: University of Minnesota Press, 2008), 95.

2. H. Gilbert Welch and William C. Black, "Overdiagnosis in Cancer," *Journal of the National Cancer Institute* 102 (2010): 605–13.

3. Ibid., 607–8.

4. Paul Goldberg, "USPSTF to Downgrade PSA Screening From 'I' to 'D'—As in 'Don't Do It,' " *The Cancer Letter* 37 (2011): 1–5.

5. Danzu Rosner, Ramez N. Bedwani, Josef Vana, Harvey W. Baker, and Gerald P. Murphy, "Noninvasive Breast Carcinoma: Results of a National Survey by the American College of Surgeons," *Annals of Surgery* 192 (1980): 139.

6. H. Gilbert Welch and William C. Black, "Using Autopsy Series to Estimate the Disease 'Reservoir' for Ductal Carcinoma in Situ of the Breast: How Much More Breast Cancer Can We Find?" *Annals of Internal Medicine* 127 (1997): 1025.

7. Virginia L. Ernster, Rachel Ballard-Barbash, William E. Barlow, Yingye Zheng, Donald L. Weaver, Gary Cutter, Bonnie C. Yankasas, Robert Rosenberg, Patricia A. Carney, Karla Kerlikowske, Stephen H. Taplin, Nicole Urban, and Berta Geller, "Detection of Ductal Carcinoma in Situ in Women Undergoing Screening Mammography," *Journal of the National Cancer Institute* 94 (2002): 1546.

8. Christopher I. Li, Janet R. Daling, and Kathleen E. Malone, "Age-Specific Incidence Rates of in Situ Breast Carcinomas by Histologic Type, 1980–2001," *Cancer Epidemiology, Biomarkers, and Prevention* 14 (2005): 1009.

9. Ernster et al., "Detection of Ductal Carcinoma," 1546.

10. Karsten J. Jørgensen, John D. Keen, and Peter C. Gøtzche, "Is Mammography Screening Justifiable Considering Its Substantial Overdiagnosis Rate and Minor Effect on Mortality?" *Radiology* 260 (2011): 623.

11. Melinda E. Sanders, Peggy A. Schuyler, William D. Dupont, and David L. Page, "The Natural History of Low-Grade Ductal Carcinoma in Situ of the Breast in Women Treated by Biopsy Only Revealed over 30 Years of Long-Term Follow-Up," *Cancer* 103 (2005): 2481.

12. Nancy N. Baxter, Beth A. Virnig, Sara B. Durham, and Todd M. Tuttle, "Trends in the Treatment of Ductal Carcinoma in Situ of the Breast," *Journal of the National Cancer Institute* 96 (2004): 443.

13. Todd M. Tuttle, Stephanie Jarosek, Elizabeth B. Habermann, Amanda Arrington, Anasooya Abraham, Todd J. Morris, and Beth A Virnig, "Increasing Rates of Contralateral Prophylactic Mastectomy among Patients with Ductal Carcinoma in Situ," *Journal of Clinical Oncology* 27 (2009): 1362–67.

14. S. W. Duffy, L. Tabar, B. Vitak, N. E. Day, R. A. Smith, H. H. T. Chen, and M. F. A. Yen, "The Relative Contributions of Screen-Detected in Situ and Invasive Breast Carcinomas in Reducing Mortality from the Disease," *European Journal of Cancer* 39 (2003): 1755.

15. Daniel B. Kopans, Robert A. Smith, and Stephen W. Duffy, "Mammographic Screening and 'Overdiagnosis,'" *Radiology* 260 (2011): 619

16. Laura Esserman and Ian Thompson, "Solving the Overdiagnosis Dilemma," *Journal of the National Cancer Institute* 102 (2010): 582.

17. Steve Graff, "Ductal Carcinoma in Situ: Should the Name Be Changed?" *Journal of the National Cancer Institute* 102 (2010): 6.

18. Esserman and Thompson, "Overdiagnosis Dilemma," 582.

19. Ann Partridge, Kristie Adloff, Emily Blood, E. Claire Dees, Carolyn Kaelin, Mehra Golshan, Jennifer Ligibel, Janet S. de Moor, Jane Weeks, Karen Emmons, and Eric Winer, "Risk Perceptions and Psychosocial Outcomes of Women with Ductal Carcinoma in Situ: Longitudinal Results from a Cohort Study," *Journal of the National Cancer Institute* 100 (2008): 248.

20. Anjali S. Kumar, Bhatia Vinona, and I. Craig Henderson, "Overdiagnosis and Overtreatment of Breast Cancer: Rates of Ductal Carcinoma in Situ; A U.S. Perspective," *Breast Cancer Research* 7 (2005): 271.

21. Joann G. Elmore, Connie Y. Nakano, Thomas D. Koepsell, Laurel M. Desnick, Carl J. D'Orsi, and David F. Ransohoff, "International Variation in Screening Mammography Interpretations in Community-Based Programs," *Journal of the National Cancer Institute* 95 (2003): 1384.

22. Agency for Healthcare Policy and Research, *Quality Determinants of Mammography* (Rockville, Md.: U.S. Department of Health and Human Services, 1994), 83.

23. Health and Consumer Protection Directorate-General, "European Guidelines for Quality Assurance in Breast Cancer Screening," 4th ed. (Luxembourg: Office for Official Publications of the European Communities, 2006), http://ec.europa.eu/health/ph_projects/2002/cancer/fp_cancer_2002_ext_guid_01.pdf (accessed August 23, 2011); NHS Cancer Screening Programmes, "Quality

Assurance Quidelines for Breast Cancer Screening-Radiology," 2nd ed. (Sheffield, UK: NHS Cancer Screening Programmes, 2011), http://www.cancerscreening. nhs.uk/breastscreen/publications/nhsbsp59.html (accessed August 23, 2011).

24. Rebecca Smith-Bindman, Philip W. Chu, Diana L. Miglioretti, Edward A. Sickles, Roger Blanks, Rachel Ballard-Barbash, Janet K. Bobo, Nancy C. Lee, Matthew G. Wallis, Julietta Patnick, and Karla Kerlikowske, "Comparison of Screening Mammography in the United States and the United Kingdom," *Journal of the American Medical Association* 290 (2003): 2129.

25. Joshua J. Fenton, Linn Abraham, Stephen H. Taplin, Berta M. Geller, Patricia A. Carney, Carl D'Orsi, JoAnn G. Elmore, and William E. Barlow, "Effectiveness of Computer-Aided Detection in Community Mammography Practice," *Journal of the National Cancer Institute* 103 (2011): 1152–61; Anoek H. J. Verchuur-Maes, Carla H. van Gils, Maurice A. A. J. van den Bosch, Peter C. De Bruin, and Paul J. van Diest, "Digital Mammography: More Microcalcifications, More Columnar Cell Lesions without Atypia," *Modern Pathology*, 24 (2011): 1191–97; Rianne de Gelder, Jacques Fracheboud, Eveline A. M. Heijnsdijk, Gerard den Heeten, André L. M. Verbeek, Mireille J. M. Broeders, Gerrit Draisma, and Harry J. de Koning, "Digital Mammography Screening: Weighing Reduced Mortality against Increased Overdiagnosis," *Preventive Medicine* 53 (2011): 134–40; Einar Vigeland, Herman Klaasen, Tor Audun Klingen, Solveig Hofvind, and Per Skaane, "Full-Field Digital Mammography Compared to Screen-Film Mammography in the Prevalent Round of a Population-Based Screening Programme: The Vestvold County Study," *European Radiology* 18 (2008): 183–91.

26. Constance D. Lehman, Constantine Gatsonis, Christiane K. Kuhl, R. Edward Hendrick, Etta D. Pisano, Lucy Hanna, Sue Peacock, Stanley F. Smazal, Daniel D. Maki, Thomas B. Julian, Elizabeth R. DePeri, David A. Bluemke, and Mitchell D. Schnall, "MRI Evaluation of the Contralateral Breast in Women with Recently Diagnosed Breast Cancer," *New England Journal of Medicine* 356 (2007): 1295–1303.

27. National Cancer Institute, "Cancer Trends Progress Report—2009/2010 Update," http://progressreport.cancer.gov/doc_detail.asp?pid=1&did=2009& chid=96&coid=929&mid=#high (accessed August 28, 2011).

28. Philippe Autier, Mathieu Boniol, Anna Gavin, and Lars Vatten, "Breast Cancer Mortality in Neighbouring European Countries with Different Levels of Screening but Similar Access to Treatment: Trend Analysis of WHO Mortality Database," *British Medical Journal* 343 (2011), http://www.ncbi.nlm.nih.gov/pmc/articles/PMC3145837/?tool=pubmed (accessed August 23, 2011).

29. Donald A. Berry, Kathleen A. Cronin, Sylvia K. Plevritis, Dennis G. Fryback, Lauren Clarke, Marvin Zelen, Jeanne S. Mendelblatt, Andrei Y. Yakovlev, Dik F. Habbema, and Eric J. Feuer, "Effect of Screening and Adjuvant Therapy on Mortality from Breast Cancer," *New England Journal of Medicine* 353 (2005): 1784.

INDEX

abortion, 9, 10

Affordable Care Act, 65, 69–70

age at screening: and American Cancer Society, 2, 20, 24, 25, 32, 33, 41, 44, 51–54, 61, 66; and American College of Radiology, 2, 33–34, 41, 51–52, 54, 61, 66; and Breast Cancer Detection Demonstration Project, 20, 21, 24, 25, 26, 29, 33, 50, 52, 56, 58; debates on, 2–3, 4, 24, 25, 32, 33, 50, 51–55, 66–69, 70, 71, 94; and false positive results, 34, 59, 64–65, 75; and high risk populations, 25, 33, 35; and HIP mammography trial, 18–19, 20, 24, 32, 52; and insurance coverage of screening mammography, 56; and menopause, 61, 70, 73, 74, 104n10; and National Cancer Institute, 24, 25, 32, 33, 52, 53–56, 57, 58, 61, 62; and National Medical Roundtable on Mammography, 34–35, 41; research on, 2–3, 33, 51–52, 54, 62,

64, 104n5; and value of screening mammography, 76

age creep, 59

AIDS Coalition to Unleash Power (ACT UP), 39

AIDS epidemic: AIDS activism, 27, 37–40, 42, 43; earliest appearance of, 26–27, 37; exponential increase in cases, 36; federal funding for, 37, 38, 40; public awareness of, 42

AIDS Treatment News, 43

Altman, Dennis, 38

American Association for Cancer Research, 23

American Cancer Society (ACS): and age at screening, 2, 20, 24, 25, 32, 33, 41, 44, 51–54, 61, 66; alliance with American College of Radiology, 23, 32, 41, 47; and breast cancer activism, 43; and breast cancer detection, 15, 19, 20–21, 23, 29, 32; and breast cancer incidence statistics, 42, 45, 48, 49; and cancer control, 6; and cervical cancer